Contents

Ken Roberts

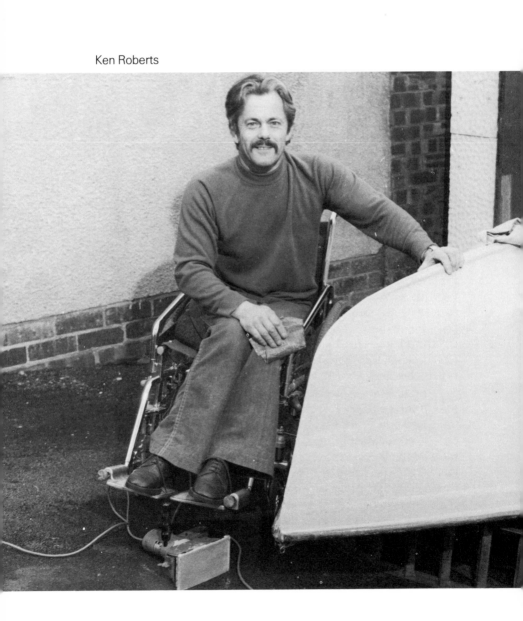

ep **Water Sports for the Disabled**

Water Sports Division:
British Sports Association for the Disabled

Water Sports for the Disabled

EP Publishing Limited

Copyright © 1983 Water Sports Division of the British Sports Association for the Disabled.

ISBN 0 7158 0864 8

First edition 1983

British Library Cataloguing in Publication Data
Water sports for the disabled.
   1. Aquatic sports—Study and teaching
   2. Physically handicapped—Recreation
   I. British Sports Association for the Disabled
      797   GV775

   ISBN 0–7158–0864–8

Published by EP Publishing Limited, Bradford Road,
East Ardsley, Wakefield, West Yorkshire, WF3 2JN,
England.

Typeset in 9/12pt Trump Mediaeval by The Word Factory,
Rossendale, Lancs.

Reproduction by Colthouse Repro Ltd.
Bournemouth, Dorset.

Printed and bound in Great Britain by Hazell Watson &
Viney Ltd., Aylesbury, Buckinghamshire, England.

Design: Douglas Martin Associates

Illustrations: Alan Sanigar

Introduction

This handbook gives some insight into how it is possible for disabled people to forget about difficulties and handicaps when they are absorbed in the demands of a sport. Not so long ago most of us thought water sports were either much too difficult or not suitable for disabled people. Fortunately a handful of far-sighted enthusiasts were bold enough to ignore convention and explore what turned out to be exciting possibilities. Soon a small group of handicapped sportsmen and women, under expert tuition and guidance, discovered that the world of water-based sports offered them increased independence and superb opportunities for extending their leisure activities.

A whole new field of recreation was now open for many disabled people who until then had thought themselves excluded.

But there could be no departure from the accepted codes of safety, and it was quickly realised that only by thorough training could disabled participants acquire that confidence which was so necessary. The standard training methods were adopted, sometimes with modifications to enable the trainee to achieve the required results, and simple adaptations to equipment were occasionally introduced. These were so successful that some of the more dedicated handicapped individuals went on to qualify as instructors, passing on their knowledge and skill to others, and far surpassing anything expected of them by those who had first set them on the path.

Throughout the early period of development, and in the succeeding phases of expansion, the governing bodies of the various sports have shown their eagerness to work with all those who shared their interest. Chief training officers have been generous with their time in helping to solve the many technical problems which have arisen, and they have encouraged their staff to join with them in making direct contact with handicapped trainees. Against this background the water recreation horizons of disabled people will continue to expand, though of course the limitations which may be imposed by individual disabilities must be recognised. Some of these are no more than inconveniences while others may appear insurmountable. But barriers have also served as a stimulus to enterprise and inventiveness. Angling, canoeing, power boating, rowing, sailing, sub-aqua diving and water skiing offer excellent opportunities for handicapped people to discover that their abilities have been underestimated by most people, often including themselves.

The greatest benefits to be derived from water sports will perhaps be experienced by disabled youngsters. Boys and girls have shown that, despite their handicaps, they often have the courage of lions. They deserve every encouragement to enable them to take part in these rewarding outdoor pursuits. In shared enjoyment of a sport, apparent differences become insignificant.

The present situation is ripe for further success. On the one hand there are numerous disabled people of all ages who are seeking new leisure outlets. On the other are the disabled 'elite', as these experts have been called, apparently possessing the almost magical ability to handle water sports equipment as though their handicaps did not exist. Stirred by their example, and by the recognition that here lies an opportunity for genuine integration between able-bodied and handicapped people such as few other sports can offer, we look forward to a period of development in which more and more disabled people will be enabled to achieve success, fulfilment and enjoyment in these ways.

Ken Roberts
Chairman, Water Sports Division of B.S.A.D.

Water Sports Division of the British Sports Association for the Disabled

In 1973 the Sports Council in England, realising the growing interest in, and the potential of, water sports for disabled people, set up an Advisory Panel comprising the governing bodies of all the sports involved, together with a number of organisations and individuals with knowledge and experience. After seven highly productive and formative years, during which the Panel established itself as a leading authority, the decision was taken to merge with the British Sports Association for the Disabled, the national co-ordinating body of sport for disabled people. A major step forward was also taken when, with the aid of a grant from the Rehabilitation and Medical Research Trust, a National Co-ordinator was appointed. His activities have already resulted in a considerable growth of knowledge, co-operation and participation in this area of sport.

The aims of the Water Sports Division of B.S.A.D., as it is now known, are:

- To co-ordinate developments concerning disabled participants in angling, canoeing, power boating, rowing, sailing, sub-aqua, water skiing and other water sports activities.
- To provide training programmes suitable for disabled people who wish to become proficient in water sports, and to guide instructors in dealing with handicapped trainees.
- To initiate research on technical aids and equipment to help disabled people enjoy water sports.
- To act as a clearing house for information and advice.

The first handbook was published in 1977, and brought under one cover the considerable expertise which existed in the various sports. The exchange of views and experiences which its production involved, and their wider dissemination, have led to many new developments. The demand for the book, both in the United Kingdom and abroad, has indicated the extent of the need it was intended to meet, and its authoritative standing has been widely recognised.

So much has happened in the intervening years in this fast-developing field that the time is now ripe for a revised and amplified edition which can take account of the many new initiatives. In the first edition, for example, little reference was made to the participation of the mentally handicapped. It is good to be able to report many successful instances where those concerned for people handicapped in this way have found that water sports can provide the same stimulating challenge, as well as an enjoyable interest. It is acknowledged that there is still much to be learned in this direction; a study is planned with a view to further research so that eventually more detailed guidance can be given. Information from those who already have experience would be much welcomed.

The Division consists of individuals, many of them disabled, who are water sports enthusiasts and representatives of the following organisations:

Amateur Rowing Association
British Canoe Union
British Sub-Aqua Club
British Water Ski Federation
British Disabled Water Ski Association
National Anglers' Council
Royal Yachting Association
British Sports Association for the Disabled
Scottish Sports Association for the Disabled
Welsh Sports Association for the Disabled

Department of Education and Science (Observer)
Sports Council (Observer)

The Division is profoundly grateful to the Rehabilitation and Medical Research Trust for their financial support. It would not be possible to mention by name all those who have contributed to this publication but we would like to record our thanks to them and especially to Isabel Anderson, Norman Croucher, Len Warren, Tony Edge, Tim Marshall, Oliver Cock, Noel O'Brien, Don Robertson, Ron Moore and Bob Bond for their particular contributions. We are grateful also to the many photographers who have so willingly allowed their work to be used.

We are also indebted to Keith Jary for his work in collating and editing the material for this revised edition. Thanks are also due to Elizabeth Dendy of the Sports Council. Her steady guidance throughout and her constant encouragement have enabled us to achieve much more than seemed possible when first we gathered together.

1. Risk and Disability

Most of the activities described in this handbook come into the category of risk sports; participation in them involves the direct possibility, however small, of death or injury. There is an element of danger in almost any activity one can think of, and everyone has the freedom to decide whether the enjoyment or pleasure derived from that activity is worth the risk involved. This is a freedom which can be exercised without restraint by the able-bodied, and there are strong arguments for ensuring that the same freedom can be enjoyed by those for whom a congenital defect, or a later accident or illness, has resulted in handicap.

To ensure that the risk is equivalent, due allowance must be made for the *extra risk* which might arise from the handicap. Limited experience, lack of experienced companions, lack of sophisticated or reliable equipment, and disability are all handicaps which are in some ways comparable. They all increase risk, so they all set limits on what can be undertaken without *undue risk*. If one or more of these elements applies to an individual it may be unwise for him to engage in certain activities, but perfectly safe for him to engage in others; the risk in long-distance ocean sailing, for example, may be too high, whereas that in less exacting trips could be quite acceptable. The experienced disabled participant may be more competent than an able-bodied novice, and the handicap in itself must not result in disabled people being needlessly denied opportunities. There are, of course, handicaps which clearly preclude participation in some sports: it would be foolhardy for someone who has epileptic seizures to go sub-aqua diving, for example.

2. Medical Considerations

Before a disabled person takes up a water sport the opinion of a general practitioner should be sought to ensure that there are no medical reasons why the sport should not be practised. The advice which follows has been prepared for the preliminary guidance of disabled people, helpers and instructors, and gives a brief description of the more common disabilities with their implications for water sports.

ANTERIOR POLIOMYELITIS (POLIO)

This is a viral infection affecting the nerves supplying various muscle groups in the body. As a result, weak muscles are produced in the region affected. The degree of paralysis varies from an isolated weakness of a shoulder or foot to a widespread weakness of a whole limb. In addition to weak muscles, the individual may be troubled by deformity of the limb due to muscle wasting and tendon contractures.

Provided the arms are strong and the individual is able to swim for a short distance, polio need not be a deterrent to water sports. Severely affected limbs may have poor blood supply, and therefore chilblains and skin ulcers may occur more easily when the limb becomes wet and cold.

Special care should be taken to protect severely affected limbs, and they should be dried carefully after exposure. Canoeing has proved particularly popular with many people suffering from polio because the limb functions required may often be within their capabilities.

CEREBRAL PALSY

A condition resulting from damage to the brain before birth or at any time during childhood. It is sometimes accompanied by mental retardation, epilepsy and emotional disorders. There are three main types of cerebral palsy and they can be basically recognised under the following headings:

Athetoid. This is marked by a dis-coordinated involuntary movement.
Spastic. This is shown by muscle spasm and exaggerated reflexes
(hyperreflexia), often with rigidity. The person may suffer from paralysis of
the body down one side, or of all four limbs to a greater or lesser degree.

Ataxic. This is shown by an inability to make rapid co-ordinated movement.

Participation in water sports for any particular individual obviously depends on the degree of disability, but particular attention should be paid to the presence of athetosis, as this could lead to sudden loss of balance in light craft.

Should a spastic individual inhale water, widespread muscle spasm may make it difficult for him to expel it. Some spastics find that the stiffness of their limbs is increased in cold water and by over-exertion; this could be brought on as a result of too much encouragement from an instructor.

SPINA BIFIDA

A failure in spinal development before birth results in the spine being divided by a cleft in the lower back instead of fusing normally. There may be an associated failure of development of the spinal cord of varying degree, resulting in weakness and wasting of the muscles of the legs and feet. As well as muscle wasting, other abnormalities such as club foot and a swollen head may occur.

These do not usually produce problems except that occasionally, to relieve the fluid retention in the head, a plastic valve is inserted below the skin at the side of the neck. Some individuals with spina bifida will also have paralysis of the nerve supply in the bladder and bowel, with consequent incontinence.

In water sports where legs are needed, such as rowing, severe cases may experience difficulty. When a valve is in place, trauma to this area should be avoided. If rowing or canoeing are contemplated, care should be taken of the skin over the buttocks and lower limbs.

There is often an associated loss of skin feeling over these areas, and breaks in the skin leading to ulcers may occur without the individual being aware of it. Good protective clothing and meticulous care of the skin are important in affected individuals.

SPINAL CORD PARALYSIS

A disease or trauma which damages the spinal cord at a certain level resulting in paralysis of the muscles that are supplied below the level of the injury. The paralysis may be floppy (*flaccid*) or stiff (*spastic*) and affect either the lower limbs (*paraplegic*) or all four limbs (*tetraplegic*).

If both legs are paralysed but the arms are not affected, they may become strong from constant use of crutches or a wheelchair, and water sports such as sailing are certainly possible. There may be a lack of sensation in the legs associated with paralysis, and the same considerations of skin protection apply as for the individual with spina bifida. Incontinence may also be a difficulty. Sudden immersion in cold water may lead to an increase in muscle spasm which could cause problems in an emergency.

AMPUTEES

Amputations may be of legs or arms, at high or low level. The type of water sport contemplated will therefore depend on the type of amputation and the amputee's competence with or without artificial limbs. There may be problems of balance if the patient has to swim unexpectedly, so assistance should always be near at hand.

Hardware such as artificial limbs and braces can prove a problem in the water and may deteriorate if it becomes wet during the course of the sport. To cope with this, some amputees wear old artificial limbs. Anyone intending to sail regularly should consider enquiring at his limb centre about artificial legs suitable for water sports.

Amputees who have lost limbs as a result of circulatory disorders should take particular care in water sports. The 'phantom limb' sensation may occur.

MULTIPLE SCLEROSIS

In this disease, of unknown origin, isolated plaques of degeneration occur throughout the nervous system, producing a variety of symptoms and signs. Perhaps the most common, and the one that may hinder the individual most, is paralysis below the waist. This paralysis may be spastic or flaccid and, as with spina bifida, incontinence may occur. There is also a loss of sensation and of balance.

A characteristic of the disease is a period of remission, often accompanied by euphoria. Some individuals may find it difficult to use their arms in the normal way. The hand sometimes trembles and is unable to carry out fine movements, which might produce problems in sailing. Occasionally the disease leads to blindness, and enquiries about sight are relevant before allowing anyone with multiple sclerosis on the water by himself. It is essential to prevent undue fatigue.

VISUAL HANDICAP

The blind and partially sighted can have problems in water sports. Those with a detached retina must avoid knocks and strenuous activity, which may prevent participation. Provided visually handicapped people are always accompanied by a sighted person, many difficulties can be overcome. The visually handicapped often have an increased sensitivity to the environment and an extra ability to concentrate which accelerates learning.

MUSCULAR DYSTROPHY

A progressive disease occurring mostly in boys, producing flaccidity and loss of muscle tone, ultimately affecting the muscles of respiration. Constant medical checks must be made and fatigue prevented. The flaccidity often makes it difficult to handle muscular dystrophy victims, and previous consultation with their general practitioner is essential.

ASTHMA

Asthmatics might contemplate water sports, depending on the severity of the asthma, but they should always be accompanied in case of emergency.

EPILEPSY

Epilepsy presents particular problems. The individual may not have had a fit for some years and be well controlled on drugs. Whether he or she should be barred from taking part in water sports is a complex question and it has been thought wise to devote a separate section to it (see p.17).

DEAFNESS

Many deaf people take part in water sports and the main problems are the possibility of giddiness and disturbance of posture.

This list of disabilities is by no means comprehensive, and if further details are required, reference can be made to other publications referred to in the Bibliography, including the *Textbook of Sport for the Disabled* (Guttman), *Guidelines for Teaching Disabled People to Swim* (Trussell), pamphlets of the National Co-ordinating Committee on Swimming for the Disabled and the Cerebral Palsy International Sports and Recreation Association, and the *Riding for the Disabled Handbook* (Riding for the Disabled Association).

Common sense and careful assessment of the physical disability will usually enable the individual and his instructor, after consultation with a doctor and/or therapist, to decide which particular water sport is possible. Detailed consideration of all the problems which may occur will not remove the risk of an emergency, and until he is extremely proficient the handicapped person should never consider going out on the water, or into the water, unaccompanied.

It is worth mentioning the help to morale in taking up a new sport, or resuming a sport experienced before an accident, and the benefits of social contact, physical well-being, and mental stimulation and relaxation. These are therapies of which any doctor would approve.

MEDICAL CONSENT FORM

It is obviously very important that those responsible for disabled people should know the extent and implications of the more common disabilities so they do not put a trainee into a potentially dangerous situation. If such a situation should arise, the organiser should know what to expect in an emergency. A disabled applicant should complete a medical form to be signed by a doctor or medical authority. An example is given in Appendix 3. The form can be adapted to suit the different physical requirements of each sport and gives the instructor and staff in charge valuable information.

3. Water Sports and Epilepsy

It is hoped that as far as possible no one with epilepsy will be needlessly excluded from the fun of water sports, nor unwisely encouraged to take part. The advice that follows is concerned not with the general risks inherent in these activities but with the additional hazards which may be directly attributed to epilepsy.

WHAT IS EPILEPSY?

An epileptic attack is due to an occasional sudden abnormal discharge from brain cells — like an electric storm in the brain. Epilepsy itself is an established tendency to recurrent fits.

Anyone can have a fit if the insult or stress to the brain is great enough. Epilepsy occurs in people of all ages, of all social backgrounds and of all levels of intellect.

Because the electrical storm can occur in any part of the brain, and the brain is responsible for all our actions and for interpreting all sensations, there can be many different types of epileptic attack, with many manifestations. However, there are three main types of attack:

Major seizures (Grand Mal)

These can be frightening, especially for anyone seeing them for the first time. The person will suddenly fall, often without warning, becoming unconscious and making involuntary convulsive movements which are sometimes vigorous. At the onset there may be a cry or strange noises, there may also be slight frothing or bubbling at the mouth, occasionally tinged with blood as a result of biting the tongue or lips. After the attack is over the person may appear confused or tired for some time.

Absences (Petit Mal)

These may be barely noticeable: they may look like day-dreaming or momentary blankness. Sometimes there is rhythmic excessive blinking. These short spells of unawareness usually last for only a few seconds. The person stops what he or she was doing.

Psychomotor fits

These attacks vary a great deal but often consist of automatic actions associated with clouding of consciousness. Often these actions are carried out in a confused manner and at the onset the person may experience various bodily sensations or emotions, such as fear. To an onlooker the person may seem to be conscious yet unable to respond during the attack, and the events of the attack are not remembered afterwards.

In some cases seizures follow a pattern of occurrence but these patterns may change and so cannot be relied on, particularly where risk sports are concerned. Warning feelings may be experienced before seizures: these may occur days or hours in advance (*prodromal* symptoms) and may include feelings of uneasiness, irritability, anxiousness or excitement. Immediately before an attack shows itself in an intense form, there may be feelings of numbness or flashes of light or one of a variety of other signs, all referred to as 'auras'. Although these auras do not always occur, and their nature may change, they can reduce the risk factor for the person, who is thereby able to alert companions or bystanders that an attack is likely.

WHAT TO DO

For a major seizure

Keep calm. Leave the person having the fit where he is, unless in danger from traffic, fire or water. Once breathing has restarted put something under the head and turn the head to one side. If nothing else is available, cradle the head in your hands. When the attack is over, allow the person to lie quietly until consciousness is regained. Make sure that he is not left alone during the period of confusion which may follow.

For other seizures

Absences and psychomotor seizures will rarely call for any action on your part, except long-term consideration for the person concerned.

WHAT NOT TO DO

- Do not be afraid, or if you are, try not to show it.
- Do not restrain convulsive movements.
- Do not ever force anything hard between the lips or teeth. Bitten tongues heal, broken teeth do not.
- Do not give anything to drink during the attack.
- Do not call a doctor unless the seizure lasts more than 15 minutes, or is followed immediately by others without the patient regaining consciousness in between.

Pairing

The system of pairing a person with epilepsy with a capable (and non-epileptic) companion who knows what to do when a seizure occurs can reduce the anxiety of instructors who are unfamiliar with this handicap, and at the same time reduce risks. 'Capable' implies that the companion could life-save in any circumstances in which the person with epilepsy might finish up. The companion should be able to recognise an attack immediately it starts and must be physically capable of supporting the person he is responsible for in deep water. Somebody should be watching both the person with epilepsy and the companion. The latter suggestion is one way of reducing the risk, provided, of course, that the person watching can assist rapidly or obtain immediate assistance.

SHOULD PEOPLE WITH EPILEPSY TAKE PART IN WATER SPORTS?

Many people with epilepsy have their attacks completely or partially controlled by anti-epileptic drugs. Some, whose seizures have been absent or have occurred only during sleep for the previous three years, can hold a private driving licence. Contrary to popular belief, therefore, people with epilepsy need not all be barred automatically from activities which become risky if consciousness lapses. Studies of swimming accidents in Hawaii and Australia show the absolute risk of drowning as a result of an epileptic attack while swimming is low; but children and adults who are also mentally handicapped, and likely to have more severe epilepsy, are at greater risk. For anyone with a history of epilepsy the most important question in the context of water sports is this: how great is the additional risk to himself, or to others, when repeated immersion in cold water may take place?

Assessment

The importance of treating each person individually cannot be over-emphasised. Before participation in water sports an *informed* medical opinion should be sought, and in each case several factors must be weighed in connection with the epilepsy, the person and the activity. The greatest danger comes from undeclared epilepsy, and in one recent case of this kind someone drowned on a canoe marathon.

The following factors should be taken into account in making an assessment:

The nature of the epilepsy:

- Whether the person has seizures or not.
- The form and severity of the seizure and the degrée of control by drugs.
- Preliminary warning indications; triggers and patterns.

The person

- Can he swim, or at least, is he able to cope in cold water with confidence?
- What previous experience has he?
- Is he likely to behave in a mature way and with common sense?

The activity

- What is the nature of the sport being considered?
- Will a lifejacket or buoyancy aid be worn?
- What supervision and instruction is available?
- Are there opportunities for pairing with an experienced person?
- How many people will be taking part and how experienced are they?
- Under what kind of weather conditions and at what time of year will the sport be practised?
- Will it be on the sea, a lake or a river, and what is the likely water temperature?
- What are the safety arrangements? Is there a safety boat available?
- What type of craft is to be used? This is particularly important in canoeing, for example.

The National Co-ordinating Committee on Swimming for the Disabled gives the following useful advice on recognising a fit in the water and dealing with it:

Watch for loss of co-ordinated movement. Some people with epilepsy continue the activity they were performing in the early stages of the attack, but their stroke becomes unco-ordinated and starts to break up. Direction becomes vague and involuntary head movements may start.

HOW CAN A FIT BE DEALT WITH?

The first priority is to keep the face above water, and it is best to approach the swimmer from behind. If it is possible, he should be towed to shallow water and his head held until the attack passes. He will do less damage to himself in the water than on land if his breathing is functioning. However, after the convulsion is over, the swimmer should be removed from the pool side. If breathing has stopped, normal resuscitation measures should be taken. Close surveillance of someone liable to major attacks is especially necessary, and familiarity with the particular type of seizure is obviously desirable on the part of the companion. Absence attacks are brief, but the swimmer may suddenly sink. The British Epilepsy Association has published a poster which describes first aid measures to be taken in case of major attacks.

Is medical assistance necessary?

No, provided resuscitation is not required, there is no injury, and one attack does not follow another without the person regaining consciousness in between (*status epilepticus*). This condition is rare, but when it does occur it is a medical emergency and help should be summoned immediately.

Lifejackets

In the event of a seizure while in the water it seems likely that a life jacket (*not* a buoyancy aid) would function normally and turn the wearer on his back, thus preventing drowning. As yet, however, there is no practical experience to confirm this, and the B.S.A.D. Water Sports Division would welcome evidence on the functioning of lifejackets in these circumstances. The risk of the tongue blocking the throat has also been suggested, and although no evidence has been found, this must for the present be regarded as a small but potentially fatal risk. Perhaps the comparison may be made with mountaineering; it is well known, for example, that falling rock can kill, yet it is still common practice to venture into areas where a certain amount of stonefall occurs, particularly in the very early morning when ice binds the rocks and so reduces the risk.

INDIVIDUAL SPORTS

When sports are considered individually guidance can be more specific, but there is room for more research.

Angling

If seizures are completely eliminated no extra precautions are required, though one could play extra safe and assume a seizure *might* occur. If seizures are possible, safety will be increased by having a capable companion nearby, and by choice of fishing sites where the person would not fall or slide into the water in the event of a seizure. When angling from a small boat the criteria are similar to those for sailing.

Sub-aqua

The policy of the British Sub-Aqua Club is that no person with a history of epilepsy should take part in this sport.

Cruising

Safety lines and lifejackets are a wise precaution in this case for anyone, and if there is any possibility of a seizure, then reliable supervision or pairing would reduce the risk. There could still be some hazards arising from seizures. Comments made previously under 'Lifejackets' (see p.21) are particularly relevant.

Rowing

The Amateur Rowing Association has knowledge of people with good seizure control who row; if the swimming definition of 'seizure free', i.e. 'one year (with) adequate blood anti-convulsant concentration' is used, the risk should be small in *warm* water. The presence of other oarsmen reduces the risk. Because oarsmen do not wear lifejackets the risk if a seizure did occur is increased.

Water skiing

If seizures are absent there is no argument against water skiing. However, if there is any possibility at all of a seizure the risk would be greatly increased and this activity is not recommended. Even in cases of minor attacks there is no certainty that the person would change direction when necessary to avoid an obstacle such as another boat, or a jetty.

Canoeing

Kayak. If a seizure leads to a capsize in this type of canoe, unconsciousness and rigidity of the body could result in the person remaining in the canoe. A lifejacket or buoyancy aid would tend to keep them pressed up under the canoe or floating on one side. Drowning would be likely. Kayak canoeing is therefore not recommended unless seizure control is total. Perhaps some people might not agree with this guidance, but in view of the indefinable degrees of extra risk involved it is felt that this activity should not be encouraged. If people do exercise their freedom of choice and canoe when they, or a companion, may have a seizure, the risk of drowning during or after a seizure cannot be ignored.

Canadian. The Canadian type of canoe is another matter. Factors to be considered are closer to those for sailing. In kayaking the possibility of a seizure should preclude the activity altogether, whereas in Canadian canoeing more precautions might be taken to deal with the outcome of a seizure, such as pairing, use of lifejacket, buoyancy aid, choice of water etc. If canoeing is some distance from the shore, thought must be given as to how, and how quickly, the person could return to the righted craft after a capsize and a seizure. For the time being, however, Canadian canoeing, though perhaps less risky than kayak canoeing, must still be considered to hold some element of risk.

Sailing

In sailing there is again the possible risk of the airway being blocked, as suggested in the paragraph dealing with lifejackets on p.21. For any sailor a lifejacket is essential. A petit mal or other form of minor seizure could lead to unexpected behaviour resulting in an accident or capsize. Careful choice of water and pairing would obviously reduce the risk.

However, it could take a long time to right the boat and get the person having a seizure on board. The danger could be further increased if the people in the water became separated from the dinghy. Safety lines and harnesses (BS 4224, or BS 4474 for children) are recommended for use on cruisers but not on small craft because in the event of a capsize, dinghy sailors should be able to fall clear.

CONCLUSION

Acknowledgement is made to the British Epilepsy Association and to the National Co-ordinating Committee on Swimming for the Disabled (see Appendix 4 p.250) for the contents of this section. The advice given is in the light of existing experience: further research is being undertaken. Both these organisations and the B.S.A.D. Water Sports Division would welcome enquiries where further information is required, and would also be glad to learn of any experience which would add to that on which their advice is now based.

4. Which Sport for You?

GUIDANCE FOR DISABLED PEOPLE

Two factors will largely govern your choice of sport: what you can manage within reasonable limits, and what sport appeals to you. Perhaps your handicap is so severe that you can only join in as a passenger or spectator; on the other hand you may find that appropriate training, adaptation of equipment and adjustment of techniques will enable you to participate more or less fully in the sport. But you will want to find out first. Before making your choice, therefore, talk to someone who understands what is involved, preferably an instructor or coach in the sport.

The Water Sports Division of B.S.A.D. will put you in touch if you do not know anyone, so write to them. Tell them about your disability. Explain that you simply want sufficient experience to find out if it is possible for you to take part. Depending on your handicap you may also need the advice and practical assistance of a physiotherapist or doctor.

The next stage might be to join a training course for disabled people or, if such a course is not available, find out from the instructor how you can best be introduced to the sport. He should know where the conditions are most suited to you and what clubs or individuals are likely to help.

There is a difference between this trial run and actually learning to canoe, sail or dive. The intention is to find out which sport is for you. There is no failure in learning in a safe situation that your balance is not good enough, or that your arms are too weak. While finding out what you can do, you will discover also whether you wish to do it. Remember that the fundamental reason for taking part in a water sport is the pleasure you will derive from it. If you do not enjoy it then look for something you do enjoy.

Undoubtedly you will experience problems and setbacks, and if at first you experience a rebuff, do not be discouraged or put off. Access and transport may be difficulties, and in addition there will be unavoidable costs. There are obvious advantages in using the shared facilities of a club or training establishment, and enthusiasm will often overcome what may appear to be insurmountable problems. Some centres and clubs are not able to cater for disabled people and some, regrettably, are reluctant to do so. But much progress has been made over the past few years, and attitudes are changing as people become more knowledgeable and understanding about the needs of the handi-capped, and about their capabilities. There are many who are willing to share the enjoyment of their sport.

However, the responsibility for choosing to take part in a sport, and for accepting the risks involved, lies largely with you; it would not be fair for adults to expect others to assume complete responsibility for them in risk sports. Many people will be willing to help in a variety of ways, but they will need your guidance on how to do this. For instance, if those helping to lift you into a boat appreciate the danger of knocking an insensitive limb, they will be far more careful and successful. People who have not had much direct contact with the disabled may be somewhat apprehensive, and need reassurance and help to overcome their fears.

So do not ignore your disability; be prepared to tell your helpers of the implications. Above all appreciate the importance of looking after yourself and keeping fit. You may have to show a lot of initiative and determination in order to take up your chosen sport, but many have already done so. Provided you really want to, you will find your opportunity.

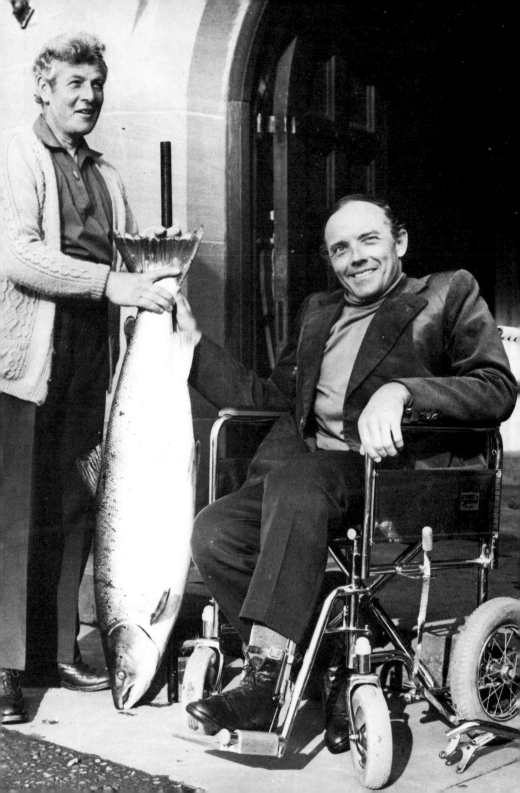

5. Angling

Angling is a very popular sport. It is often said that more people follow it as a hobby than any other recreational activity. Certainly it is one in which both young and old can take part without distinction, and in which the equipment and techniques can be very simple and rudimentary or highly sophisticated. It is also, fortunately, a sport in which the disabled person can often participate on equal terms with the able-bodied. It can be practised purely for enjoyment and pleasure with no thought of competition, or its adherents can measure their skill against each other in matches. There are three types of angling: game fishing for salmon, trout and sea trout; coarse fishing for all other species of freshwater fish; and sea fishing. All of them can be enjoyed from bank, shore or boat.

The techniques for each branch vary, as does the tackle required, but disabled anglers with the ability to hold a rod by some means or other can participate, provided that there is access to the water.

COARSE FISHING

Coarse fishing, usually the most leisurely form of angling, is especially suitable for the handicapped, practised as it is on rivers, lakes and ponds. It is not essential to be constantly on the move. The need to manipulate tackle can be quite small, and casting, using the fixed-spool reel, is relatively easy for most disabled anglers. Where problems of handling do arise, the use of a fishing pole can often overcome them.

GAME FISHING

Because of the special requirements for casting, which may require considerable effort, game fishing can be more difficult for disabled anglers, who need to have full use of one arm.

Boat fishing for trout is popular, and can be simplified by the use of special swivelling chairs with removable backs and adjustable footrests. The Scottish Committee for the Promotion of Angling for the Disabled have designed these, and they are manufactured by Buccleuch Engineering Ltd (see Appendix 4 p.250 for address).

SEA FISHING

Sea fishing may be from the beach, a pier or a boat. For wheelchair anglers beach fishing has obvious difficulties if there is no hard standing, but the problems of wheeling on sand and small stones can be overcome by using mobile tracks. The ability to cast is, however, necessary. Pier and boat fishing can be enjoyed from a sitting position. In both beach and pier fishing the disabled angler will need to be able to cast, but in boat fishing a simple drop line can be used with good effect and he can manage without any distance casting.

TACKLE

Because of the physical requirements, coarse and sea fishing appear to offer the best opportunities for most disabled people. Special tackle is needed for both branches of the sport, and usually bait, which needs to be purchased fresh. Basic tackle includes rods, reels, lines and nets, with recurring items such as hooks, floats, shot, bait etc.

A great deal can be spent on equipment and the range is very wide, but an angler can be fitted out at quite modest cost. Where only a pole is used the cost can be reduced even further. Rod kits are available and can perhaps be made at home by the angler himself. For some, this will be an added attraction to the sport, as well as reducing the expense.

Sea fishing tackle can usually be hired from professional boatmen, but coarse fishing tackle is not generally hired, although clubs which already have disabled members may be able to help.

PHYSICAL REQUIREMENTS

Having looked at the three types of angling, it is as well to look at the actual requirements of the sport.

Angling seems to cater for a greater range of disabilities than any other sport. Ideally, the angler should have the use of his arms and be sighted, but even these capabilities are by no means essential.

Those who are sighted and have some use of their arms can take part in the normal angling courses which are at present provided throughout the country. Special courses can be arranged for blind people where there is a demand. Preferably there should be one instructor to each pupil.

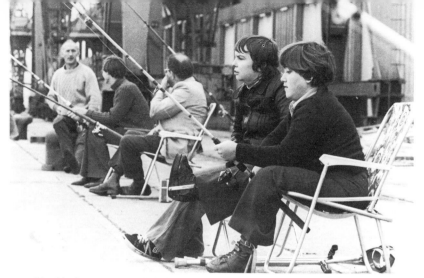

Disabled youngsters fish from the jetty.

A legless angler enjoys a day by the river. Note the shored bank against erosion.

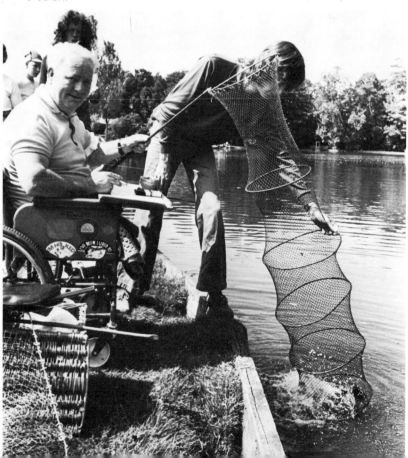

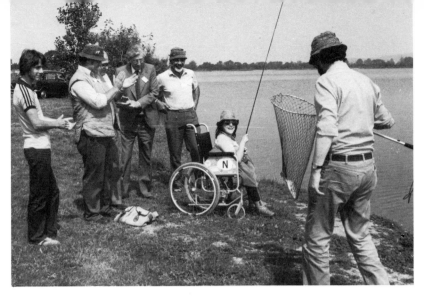

Her first catch. The level bank allows the chair to be used safely.

Bruno is a spastic unable to handle rod or reels, so his ingenious father clamped the rod to the wheelchair and fixed a reel to the electric-powered back axle which Bruno controls with his foot.

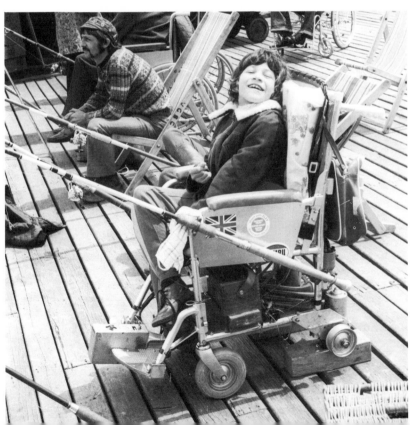

MODIFICATIONS OF EQUIPMENT AND TECHNIQUE

Rods and reels are, of course, designed for particular purposes, so selection must be based on the type of angling to be practised. The choice may well be influenced by the individual's interest, but also by his physical limitations. An instructor will be able to give advice on what kind of equipment is best suited to the disabled person and the aspect of the sport he has chosen. For example, a blind angler might very well find that ledger fishing, in which an audible bite indicator can be used, would be the best method for him.

However, there is often little need to adapt existing angling equipment, and where adaptation is required it will not alter the basic design or function. Anglers who have full use of their arms can use equipment without modification, but those using wheelchairs may require special seats for boat fishing, such as those developed in Scotland for game anglers. Anglers with restricted use of an arm will need special equipment, particularly in game fishing.

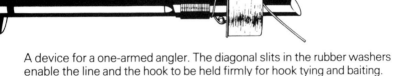

A device for a one-armed angler. The diagonal slits in the rubber washers enable the line and the hook to be held firmly for hook tying and baiting.

The 'Balcombe' landing net. Pulling on the ropes will close the net, thus trapping the fish before the angler attempts to lift them out of the water.

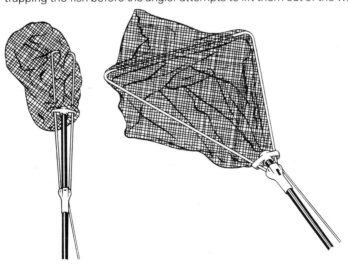

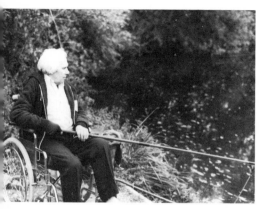 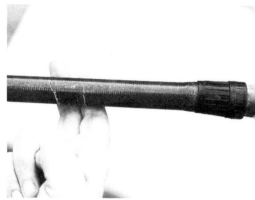

Left: Ken has severe arthritis but he fishes with a pole which requires no reel.
Right: The end of the pole is weighted with lead so that the point of balance is at the spot where it is held.

Left: Totally blind as well as having no hands, this angler holds the rod in a butt holder and with a ring over the right forearm, feeding the line over the left forearm.
Right: The large plastic disc on the inside of the reel handle enables an angler with very little grip to reel in a fish. The adaptable shoulder sling takes most of the rod weight.

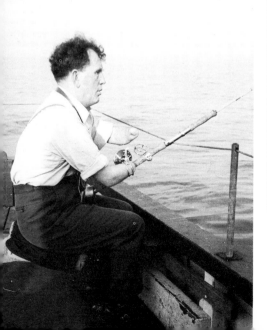 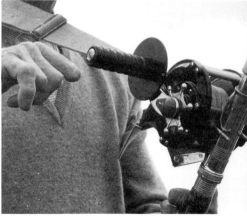

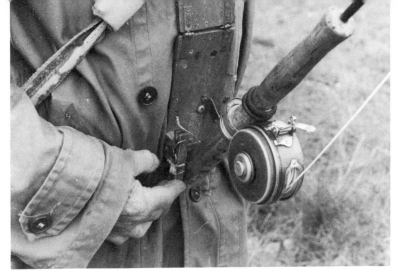

One-armed fly fisherman using automatic retrieve reel. The rod holder is mounted on a harness and the angle can be adjusted by ratchet.
The clothes peg holds the fly for changing.

The 'Mitchell' hook holder and disgorger for those with a poor grip. This can be locked in the closed position by using the retaining slot. The hook remains fixed when the grip is released.

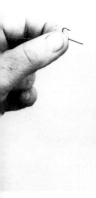
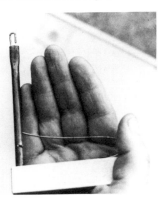
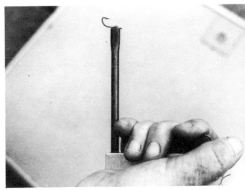

The 'Twigg' bait and hook holder for one-armed anglers. The jaws are opened by pressure of the heel of the hand to grip the hook before baiting. A foot-operated version is also available.

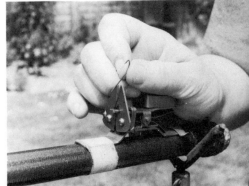

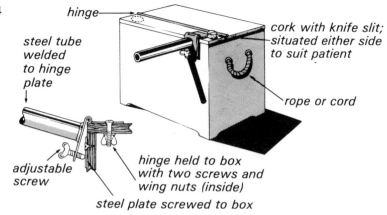

hinge

steel tube welded to hinge plate

cork with knife slit; situated either side to suit patient

rope or cord

adjustable screw

hinge held to box with two screws and wing nuts (inside)

steel plate screwed to box

Combined fishing stool and storage box with adjustable rod holder.

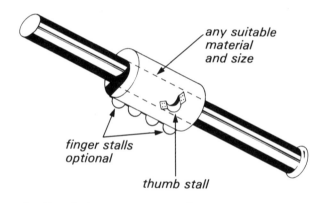

any suitable material and size

finger stalls optional

thumb stall

Enlarged rod handle to overcome poor grip.

Rod support for angler with weak grip, made of metal with plastic covering and secured by 'velcro' fastener.

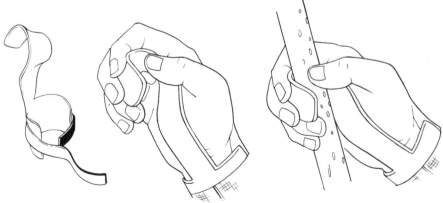

The ball attached to a conventional reel handle with finger or thumb stall helps to compensate for a weak grip.

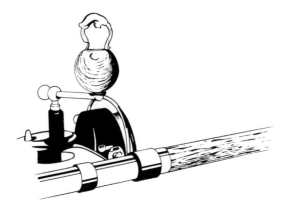

SAFETY

Any angler using a boat must observe the normal safety requirements expected of a competent boatman, including the use of a suitable lifejacket. (See 'Lifejackets and Buoyancy Aids' p.207.) He should also be able to swim or to survive in the water by keeping afloat. Anglers who have poor trunk balance need a seat with good arm rests. A safety belt can also be used, but it must have a quick release.

A crane hoist has been designed to assist those confined to chairs in boarding small boats, while on some larger vessels the individual can wheel up the gangplank. When a vessel is boarded, the boat must always be securely moored and adequate helpers must always be available.

On shore the disabled angler must be very careful when he is fishing from a position which does not provide some type of rail or fence, such as one might find on piers and in lock areas. If he is in a wheelchair he must remember that most surfaces, including grass, offer little or no grip when they are wet, and he should avoid any site with a slope towards the water. A stop block for the rear wheels is a useful item of equipment to include.

INSTRUCTION

Although the basic instruction for the disabled will not materially differ from that given to anyone else, the teacher will need to assess the disability of each individual and the limitations it is likely to impose on his movement

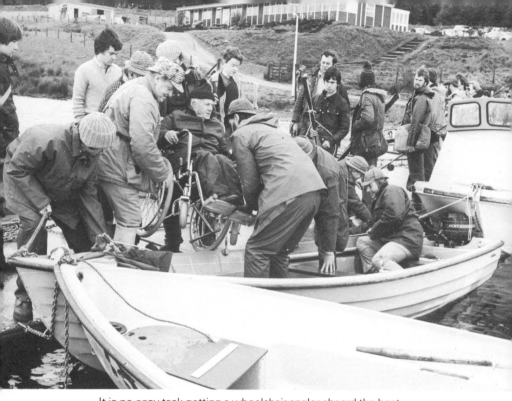

It is no easy task getting a wheelchair angler aboard the boat . . .

. . . but it can be done.

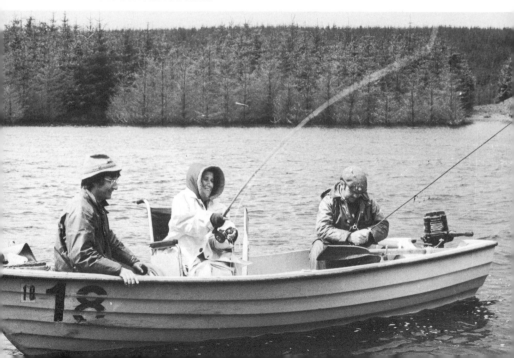

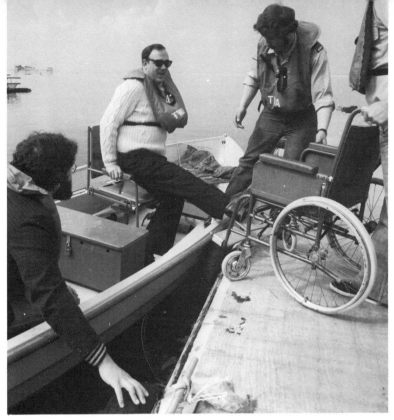

Transfer to the Buccleuch seat installed aboard is less difficult.

The seat can be pivoted to the desired angle.

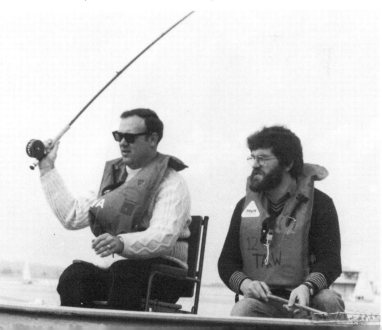

and his ability to perform the normal angling techniques. He will try to find a method of angling best suited to him and look at modifications of equipment and situations which will help to overcome the difficulties involved. The greater the disabilities, the smaller the number of students an instructor can successfully teach. It is often not realised just how much space is required by those in wheelchairs, and when classes are arranged indoors it may be necessary to use a hall rather than a normal classroom.

Instruction in casting outdoors.

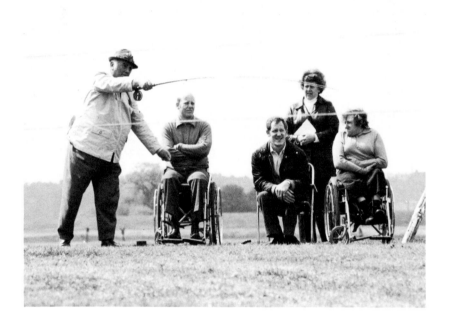

ANGLING FACILITIES FOR THE HANDICAPPED FISHERMAN

In providing facilities for the handicapped angler it is necessary to take certain requirements into consideration.

All disabled anglers require a flat surface from which to fish; it may be natural or artificial. Whatever it is, it should not slope towards the water.

For the handicapped angler confined to a chair, or the disabled person

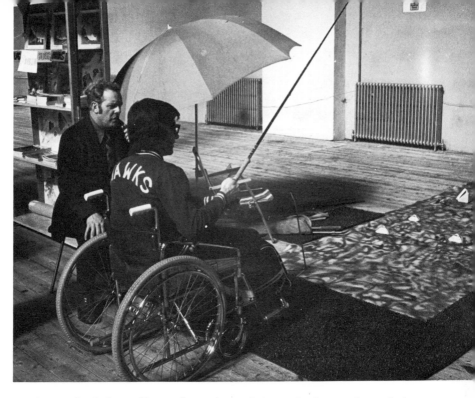

Instruction indoors. Plenty of room is needed to make the practice realistic.

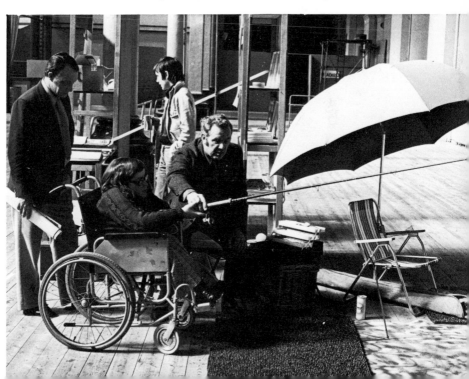

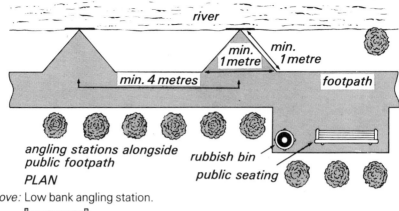

angling stations alongside
public footpath

rubbish bin

public seating

PLAN

Above: Low bank angling station.

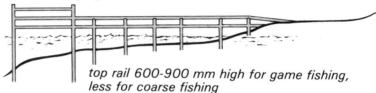

top rail 600-900 mm high for game fishing,
less for coarse fishing

Above: Angling platform in shallow water.

Below: Steep bank: access by sloping path.

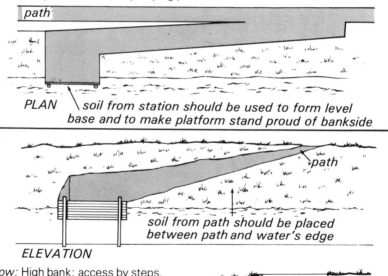

PLAN soil from station should be used to form level
base and to make platform stand proud of bankside

soil from path should be placed
between path and water's edge

ELEVATION

Below: High bank: access by steps.

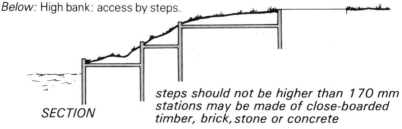

steps should not be higher than 170 mm
stations may be made of close-boarded
SECTION timber, brick, stone or concrete

who uses a stick or crutch in order to walk, a firm path and a fishing platform or station are required. These ought to be constructed of tarmac or concrete, the latter of course being more durable.

These are the basic requirements. There are, however, other refinements which should be considered and ought to be included if circumstances permit. They are listed roughly in order of priority.

Game and Coarse Fishing

The ground level should be as close to the water level as conditions permit. There should be no undercutting of the bank by erosion. Parking space for vehicles should be as close to the stations as possible. Topsoil removed from the path and fishing stations should be placed on the bank between each angling platform to raise the ground. Toilets should be near at hand and accessible, with cubicles wide enough to take wheelchairs and opening outwards. A hedge or fence along the path will provide a wind-break and cover. The disabled angler should not be separated from other anglers and there should be some provision for his family.

Sea Fishing

Access to boats and piers presents the greatest problems, and local conditions should be checked before such facilities are used by disabled people. Facilities will need to be adapted for differing venues, and expert advice should be sought before they are installed. The construction at an angling site of perhaps two or three platforms for those who are chairbound would greatly assist a section of the angling fraternity which, until now, has been sadly neglected.

Platforms along a low level bank. Note the stop board and the fixing rings for the wheelchair.

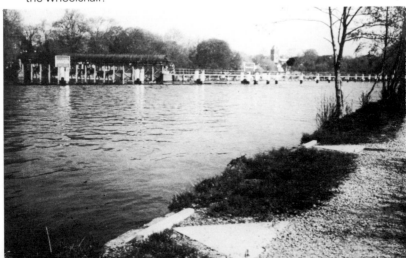

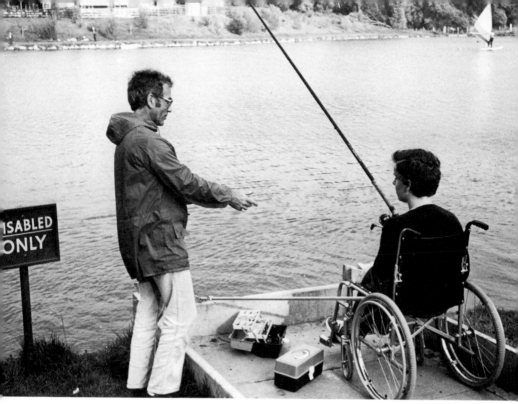

A fishing lesson for a spina bifida youngster. Note the platform built on a bank subject to erosion.

Wheelchair access to jetty over shallow bank. The platform is sturdy and gives a good position for casting.

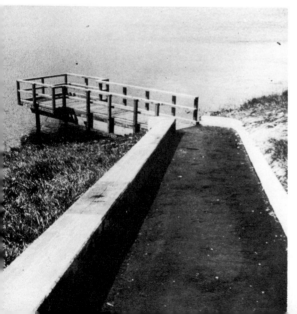

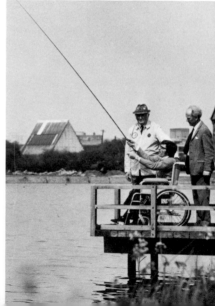

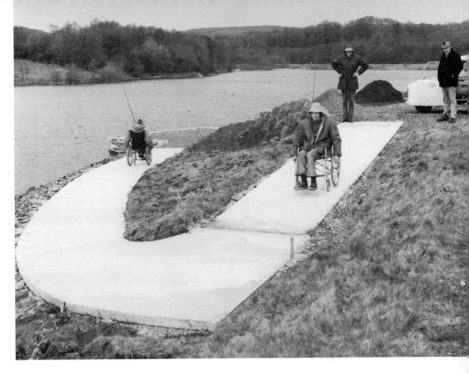

The approach overcomes the steep gradient to the shore of a reservoir which has a fluctuating water level.

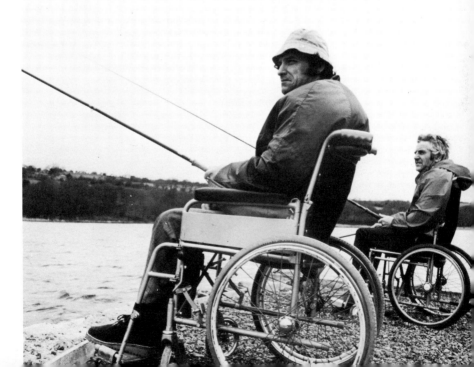

Guides to facilities

The National Anglers' Council has produced a comprehensive booklet entitled *Guide to Fishing Facilities for Disabled Anglers*, listing over one hundred fishing sites (coarse, sea and game) in England and Wales where both non-ambulant and ambulant anglers may fish. Details of each site include location, officials to contact, species of fish available, parking and shelter facilities.

The book is also a valuable source of information on special equipment, manufactured products and useful names and addresses for reference. It provides a report on a special Conference for Disabled Anglers held in London. (See Bibliography, p.250.)

Three films, entitled *Able to Fish*, dealing with coarse angling, game fishing and sea angling for disabled people have been produced by the Disabled Living Foundation, with co-operation from the National Anglers' Council. They are of equal interest to able-bodied anglers, organisations concerned with the welfare of handicapped people, and authorities with responsibility for making water available for leisure purposes. In each of the three branches of the sport, the films illustrate the problems of availability of angling waters and of access; the handling of tackle; the kinds of special aids and where they can be obtained; protective clothing; and the acquisition of practical knowledge of the pastime. There are numerous examples of disabled anglers who, by simple adaptation of equipment or the provision of specially planned facilities, have been enabled to enjoy their sport alongside their able-bodied friends. (See Bibliography, p.250, for details.)

John at the National Championship.

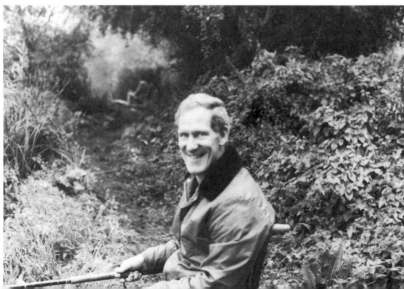

'John was 27 years of age and a severe hemiplegic who was able to move only slowly with the aid of calipers and two walking sticks. He lived with his parents; his older brothers and sisters had married and left home. He was shy and withdrawn, and the only time he went out was to his factory job as an instrument worker.

By a subterfuge an elderly neighbour, who was also handicapped but interested in angling, got John to attend angling classes for the handicapped. He quickly developed an interest and attended regularly, starting first on coarse fishing and then taking up game fishing as well. He also began to make his own floats and flies.

After a while John became secretary of a Physically Handicapped/ Able-Bodied (P.H.A.B.) type angling club and also club representative on a social committee. He has now bought an adapted motor car and regularly competes in local, regional and national competitions.

The contacts he has now made with other members of the community, both able-bodied and handicapped, have encouraged him to take part in other types of sport and in social events.

When asked about the change in his life he replied, "I damn well wasted twenty-seven years, but I am going to make up for it . . ."'

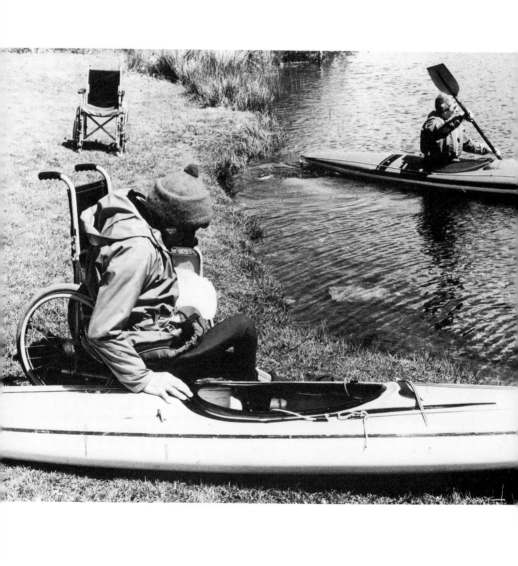

6. Canoeing

Canoeing is a very varied sport and can range from paddling gently around a lake to sliding adventurously down a rapid river, or from sprinting in the Olympics to racing over long distances. A canoeist may go to sea, either running along the shore, or venturing well out with a reliable compass. If he is interested in natural history, then the canoe will be an ideal way of studying marine or river life. Freedom and variety make canoeing an enjoyable, peaceful and relaxing activity. Anyone good with his hands can make his own canoe. It is a light craft which can easily be transported from one stretch of water to another.

Sprinting with canoes is an Olympic competition, and marathon racing of upwards of 5 kilometres (3 miles) is regarded as the cross-country form of the competition. Wild water racing has world championships. This involves racing down a rapid river. Slalom, where a canoeist has to weave his way through 'gates' made of two poles slung over a rapid, progressing from gate to gate from start to finish, is also a world championship event and has been an Olympic activity.

Sailing canoeing has the oldest cup in the world for single-handed sailing vessels, the New York Cup, an international trophy for clubs which was first awarded in 1886. Canoe surfing is a very exciting form of competition. Canoe polo is usually played in a swimming pool, using a special form of canoe.

Instructions in the pool: getting into the canoe with the instructor in the water.

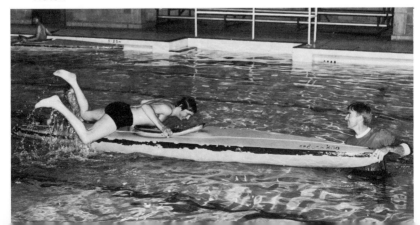

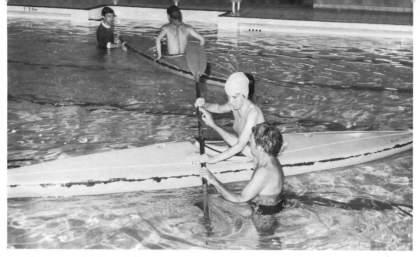
Instructor in the pool.

BRITISH CANOE UNION

The governing body of the sport in Britain, the British Canoe Union, wholeheartedly supports the participation of disabled people in canoeing, and encourages its members and particularly those involved in coaching to this end. Most of the organisation of canoeing is done through clubs, which will be found spread throughout the country. They cater for a variety of canoeists, and while some specialise in the competitive aspects of the sport, others are more interested in its purely recreational aspects. Disabled people should find themselves made welcome in most clubs, which will be prepared to help with instruction and advice on any special equipment that may be needed. Sometimes special groups are formed. An approach to the B.C.U. can often put the disabled person in touch with a suitable club or group in his area.

PHYSICAL REQUIREMENTS

The first essential for every canoeist is to be able to swim. This usually implies moving a measurable distance through the water, but the minimum requirements for the safety of a canoeist in an organised group are to be able to float with confidence after capsizing, and to come safely out of the canoe. Severely handicapped people sometimes find it difficult to achieve the normal requirement to swim 50 metres, but this should not prevent them from taking part provided that the extra supervision needed to preserve a reasonable standard of safety is available. The other physical requirements are the ability to sit up, reasonable balance, and the ability to use both arms and hands. There is no need to have use of the legs. One world championship class slalom competitor had only one leg!

Many disabled people can take part in canoeing in one form or another.

Those with polio have found it a sport they can enjoy; so have some people with cerebral palsy who have normal use of their arms. Paraplegics, even those with quite high lesions, can manage quite well, though in some cases a back rest is needed to provide the necessary support.

Blind people often paddle in the front of a two-seater canoe while those with limited vision may use a single-seater and have somebody just ahead to lead the way. A few totally blind people manage this way too. Deaf people enjoy the sport, but a sense of balance is necessary. A canoe tips easily, so it is essential to be able to keep it the right way up, at least for most of the time!

People with any weakness of the back muscles soon become tired on a long trip. It is unwise, also, for those who wear metal calipers or artificial legs to use them while canoeing, since they will be a hindrance in the water. They can be taken off and left on the bank if it is intended to return to the same point. On a short river tour, they can be put in waterproof bags and stowed below deck. In this way they are safe and easily to hand when wanted. (Suitability of cosmetic calipers for water sports has not yet been fully investigated.)

Epilepsy should not necessarily prevent someone from taking up canoeing. The frequency and severity of attacks, and the degree of control achieved by drug therapy, should be taken into account. The instructors may well need to watch closely for likely symptoms, and have the skill to deal with an attack should one occur. (See 'Water Sports and Epilepsy', p.17.)

EQUIPMENT

There are two basic types of canoe. The Eskimo type *kayak* is a decked-in craft with a round or oval cockpit in which the canoeist sits. He uses a paddle with two blades. The Indian type, or *Canadian* canoe, is open on the top, with little or no deck. The canoeist either sits or kneels and uses a paddle with a blade at one end only. In the kayak the sitting position is virtually at water-line level with the legs out in front under the deck, whereas in a Canadian the canoeist sits 200-250 millimetres (8-10 inches) above the floor, as though on a low chair. From the point of view of balance and technique these are two very different styles of canoeing. It is worthwhile to try both of them.

There are many variations on these two types of canoe, and this is another reason to go to the nearest club and find out what suits best. Especially where paralysis of the legs is involved, a kayak should have a roomy cockpit. Width is another feature to look for if balance is a problem. In general the broader the canoe the more stable it is, and the less likelihood there is of getting wet, or at least of getting wet quite so often. The Caranoe has a large cockpit and great stability, and has been found particularly suitable

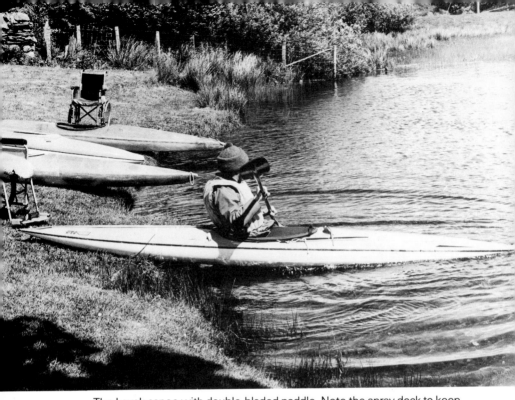

The kayak canoe with double-bladed paddle. Note the spray deck to keep the lower limbs dry.

Two disabled people paddle a Canadian canoe on a canal expedition. Single-bladed paddles and more room.

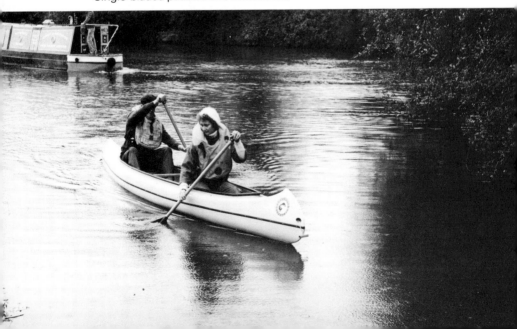

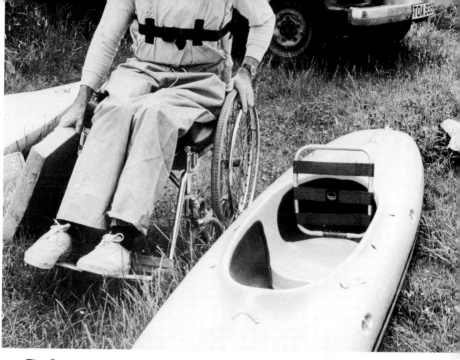

The Caranoe has a broad beam and roomier cockpit. The backrest gives support.

A well-placed cushion eases entry.

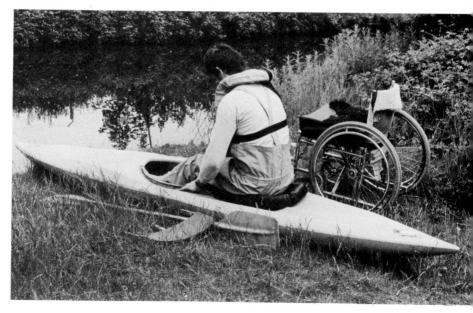

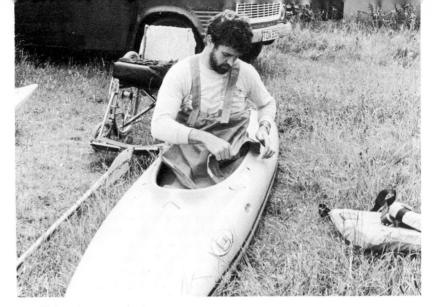

Fixing the spray deck.

Sharp edges around the cockpit and seat can cause injury.

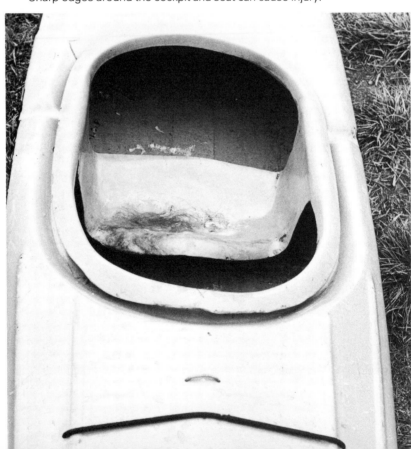

for some types of disability. Modifications to canoes to suit individual disabled people have been made by the manufacturers. (See Appendix 4, p.250.)

Many disabled people find they can use a kayak or a Canadian canoe without complications, while others need a backrest or some sort of strapping to hold them into the canoe in some way. The individual adaptations obviously reflect the particular disability and the type of craft being used, but a few general rules can be laid down. One concerns being strapped. This should never be done before the canoeist has become quite proficient. It is essential that he should practise releasing himself quickly after a capsize. He should do it under controlled conditions in a swimming pool, before he has any need to do it in earnest on a trip.

Paralysis of a limb is usually accompanied by poor circulation. There is also the danger of injuries going unnoticed because of the lack of pain, and a subsequent risk of infection. An extra cushion may also be useful in preventing pressure sores. To ensure protection the cockpit should be free from cracks, and any sharp edges should be covered with adhesive tape or neoprene. Sores may be caused by scraping, especially in glass fibre canoes. Some people find wet suits desirable because as well as keeping the body warm they help to prevent bruising. At the least any susceptible limbs should be protected with trousers, socks and plimsolls, and conventional windproof clothing should be used. In some cases it would be advisable to make a special neoprene protection for a rudimentary limb. It is foolish to be uncomfortable when there is no need. (See 'Protective Clothing', Appendix 2, p.246.)

It is not always easy to hire canoes, even when standard equipment is required. In the first place, however, equipment may often be borrowed from a helpful club. As suggested, a modest handyman may be able to build the canoe himself, much to his own satisfaction and at a saving of about half the cost of normal purchase. Local clubs often have facilities for this.

A kayak will be equipped with a spray-deck. This is a sort of rubberised skirt with an elasticated top and bottom. The top is secured around the waist and the bottom is stretched round the rim of the cockpit to stop water coming in. The legs are thus kept fairly dry and warm.

Blind people sometimes find unfeathered blades less confusing in the early stages. Ovalled looms with a taped-on mark where the hand grips the paddle will help to indicate the correct angle of the blade.

Feathered blades require flexing of the wrist that can be too demanding for anyone with a weak grip; again, unfeathered blades can help. Another alternative is a thin loom and extra-light paddle, which can have custom-made hand grips taped on. Mitts which can be held in position on the loom by using velcro may also be useful. Amputees may find Canadian blades easier to handle. An extra-long unfeathered paddle tucked under the armpits may enable a person with only rudimentary limbs to perform a satisfactory paddling stroke by moving the trunk.

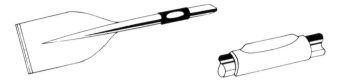

Paddle with taped-on mark to indicate the blade angle.

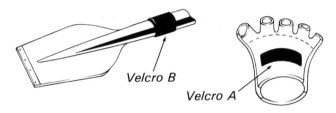

Velcro B

Velcro A

Velcro mitts or paddle ring can help those with weak grip to hold the paddle.

TECHNIQUES

The basic skills of canoeing are not difficult to learn, given reasonable balance and good arms and hands, though it is strongly recommended that a qualified instructor undertakes the teaching. The basic skills are best taught in the highly controlled situation of a swimming pool, where it is warm and the instructor can stand in the water.

In the kayak it is possible to do the 'Eskimo roll'. This involves tipping the canoe over sideways, going right underneath the canoe, and coming up again the other side. If this technique can be learned it should be possible to right the canoe in the event of a capsize, and thus avoid having to rely on other people to carry out a rescue. However, not everyone can learn to do an Eskimo roll. It will depend to some extent on the nature of their disability. If it cannot be mastered there are other drills which will facilitate rescue and the rescue of others.

Canadian canoeing is relatively uncommon in Britain, where the kayak is the more usual form of canoe. For some types of disability, however, it has distinct advantages over the kayak. Firstly, if difficulty is experienced in wriggling down into the relatively small space of a kayak cockpit, or in getting out in case of a capsize, this will be much less of a problem in an open

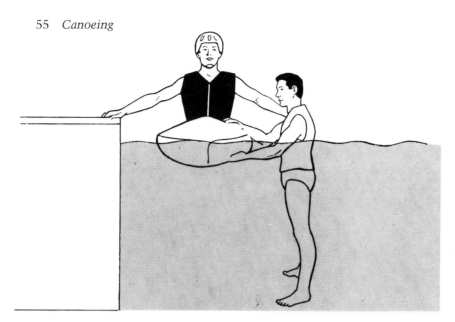

Confidence can be built up if the instructor stands in the water and holds the canoe to prevent a capsize.

Norwegian design for canoe and boathouse with floating dock and sling for disabled canoeists.

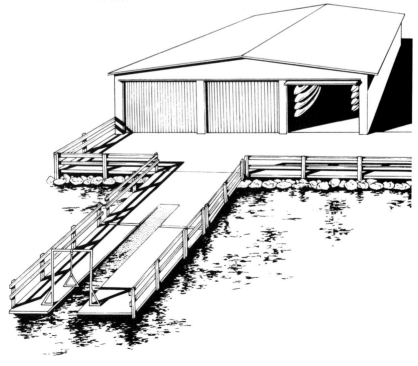

Canadian canoe. Secondly, it is more usual for two people to paddle a Canadian, and the presence of a second person can help to stabilise the boat. Thirdly, there is much more space for carrying things in a Canadian, so that if the canoeist intends to go out for more than a day it is easier to carry all the equipment needed. It is even possible to fold up a wheelchair and take it along. River canoe-camping holidays using Canadian canoes are now organised, and although these trips are not designed specifically for disabled people, it may be possible for people with certain disabilities to go on them.

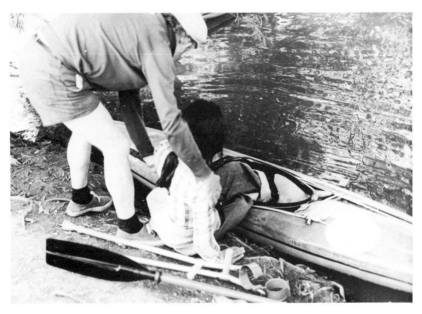

A helping hand to enter, with the kayak in the water.

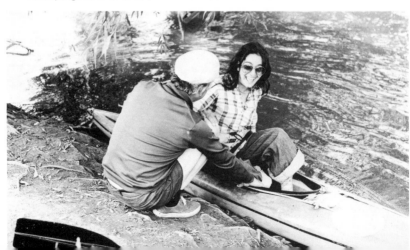

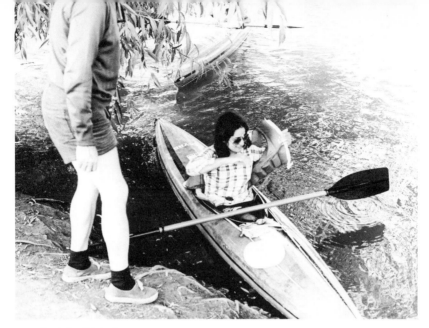

And the lifejacket.

A Norwegian paraplegic canoeist using a floating dock and sling to enter his canoe.

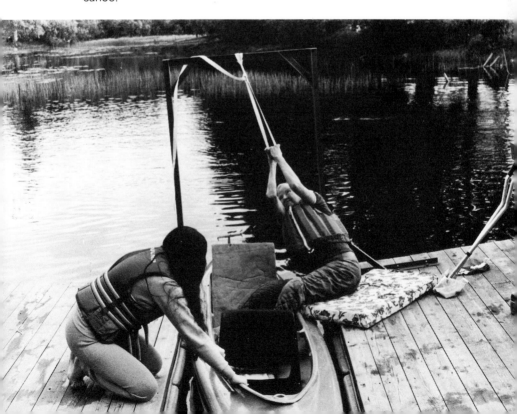

SAFETY

The need to be able to swim has already been mentioned. How far is not very important. But water confidence is. The safe canoeist will not mind being under water for a few moments when he capsizes. This is more important than being able to swim a long distance. Most people are nervous at first, but as knowledge and understanding grow, so they gain confidence. Canoeing has a good accident record.

Some form of lifejacket or buoyancy aid should always be worn. One with two stages of buoyancy, such as that approved for the sport with the British Standard Kitemark, is best. The lower stage, with about 6 kilograms (13 pounds) buoyancy helps the canoeist to swim comfortably, while the higher inflatable stage enables him to rest comfortably as he awaits rescue. However, it is very important to try out the lifejacket inflated in controlled conditions to ensure that it will cause the body to float face upwards in the event of a capsize.

Canoeing should never be done alone. There should always be at least one other experienced person, in another canoe, near to hand, so that help is available if the need arises.

Quick release of strap for an experienced paraplegic canoeist.

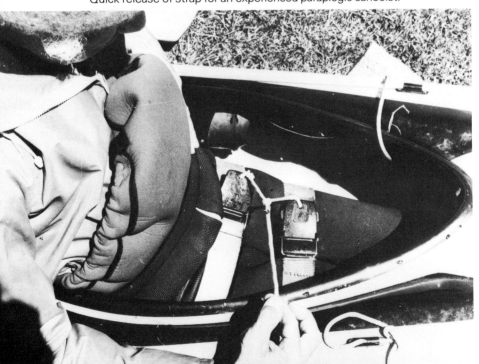

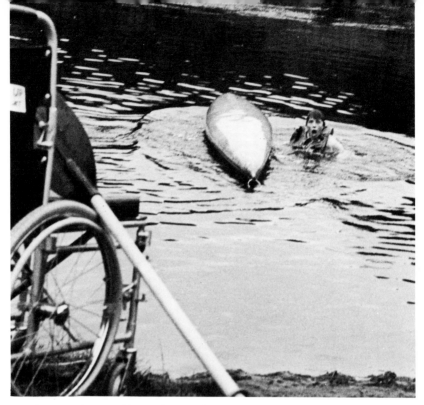

Jane, a 15-year-old spastic, practises capsize drill.

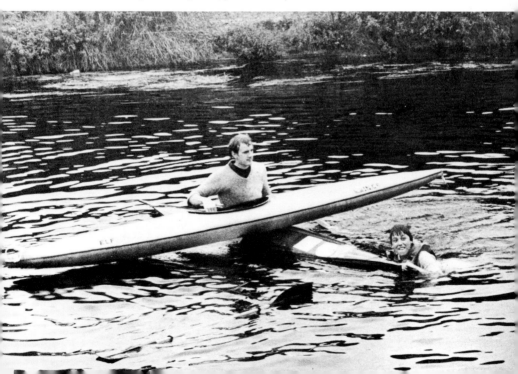

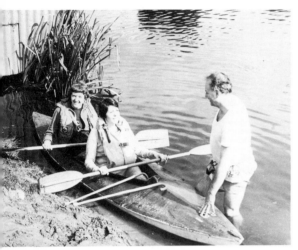

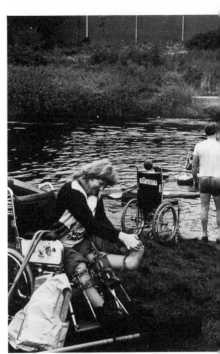

Left: Doubling up for safety. Helen (in front) has rheumatoid arthritis and is a complete beginner.

Right: Mary takes her calipers off before she goes afloat.

COURSES

Although instruction courses at various levels are held all over the country, it is worth re-emphasising that it is best to learn at a club. But if this is not possible there are many centres which run suitable courses. The Sports Council organises courses at the Plas y Brenin National Centre for Mountain Activities in Wales, and at the Bisham Abbey National Recreational Centre in Buckinghamshire. Courses are also organised in Scotland and Northern Ireland by the respective Sports Councils. The British Canoe Union will provide information about courses being run in the United Kingdom through its area and local coaching organisers, and also advise on suitable clubs in the vicinity.

To sum up, the sport of canoeing is not one which needs great adaptations for people who are disabled. They should be able to use ordinary equipment without any major modifications and play an active part in the sport like any other enthusiast.

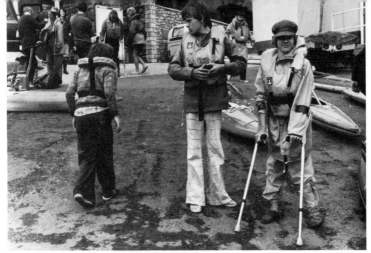

Preparing for a canoeing trip on the river Tamar.

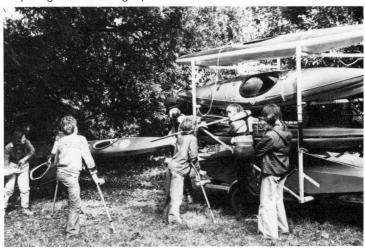

Helping to load the trailer.

Some friendly help before going afloat.

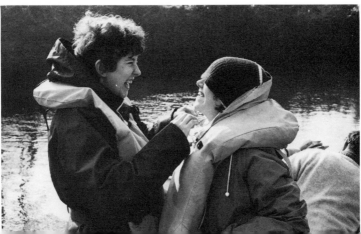

BLIND PEOPLE LEARN TO CANOE

The Poseidon Canoe Club of Mitcham in Surrey was asked by the Social Services Department if they could teach canoeing to blind people. They had no experience but received lots of advice, some of which was helpful, and some rather less so. It proved a rewarding and exciting adventure with much learned on both sides as these extracts from a fuller account by the Club Secretary indicate:

'We were fortunate in having a two-hour stint in the local swimming baths one evening a week in the summer. We had this sort of protective idea that blind people must be fragile. How little we knew.

Another illusion we had was that they were talking about youngsters. They weren't. They meant mature adults, some of them anything but young.

We started with one person. We learned about their trust in us as the "experts" which we considered to be misplaced, but daren't admit, and their aural discrimination which made nonsense of noise problems. We found that capsizing did not dismay them as it used to dismay some of us.

The first problem was paddles. We supplied straight but feathered blades. How to place the blades in the correct attitude in the water? A locating device was called for. It turned out to be a bit of stick taped on to the shaft. From there it was pretty straightforward. Paddling forward, backward, stopping, turning, support strokes etc.

We learned that there are all kinds of visual handicaps. We had someone who could see straight ahead but had no peripheral vision; someone who could see all round but not straight ahead; people who lost their sight late in life; people who were blind from birth. We soon realised that it was not a matter of type of handicap at all. It was a question of personal relationships.

Eventually we passed from swimming pool to open water — our local lake — and we returned to the signalling business. No real problem. Follow-my-leader with a sighted leader singing at the top of his voice, or a transistor on the leader's deck. But the real key to success was that each visually handicapped person had, somewhere nearby, a sighted companion whose voice they knew.

But technique is only a means to other achievements. We already had a scheme of paddling downstream on the Thames with an overnight stop at an inn. We decided to do the same with our blind friends using both double and single canoes. We launched the double with sighted

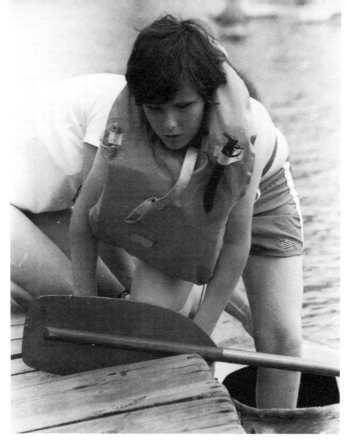

A young blind canoeist. The approved lifejacket has inherent buoyancy and can be further inflated.

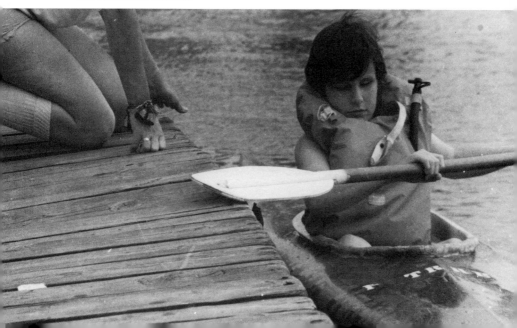

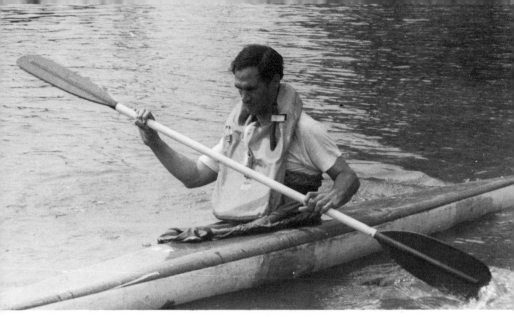

A blind canoeist practises in a kayak on a slow-moving river.

guides and single-seater canoe support. Locks to negotiate, river traffic to avoid in a glorious weekend of Indian summer.

The one-to-one relationship of sighted guide and blind paddler introduced us to a new world where the important things were hearing, smell and touch. We had to become describers and interpreters of the scene. With running commentary we could become proxy eyes. It is a fact that our sight of a kingfisher excited them more than it did us, and some of them had never seen one, ever, and never will. The sensation of floating downwards in an emptying lock, feeling the support chain running through the hands, the sounds of the water rushing out, the cheerful friendliness of the lock-keepers, boat owners and everyone else, things we took for granted, were now focused for us through their lack of vision. Shooting an easy weir became a matter of high excitement.

Peter came. He is at a residential school but comes to us usually in the holidays. As our youngest colleague and quickest learner he had already taught us some amazing things. For example he can do a still water slalom course with a minimum of direction, apparently sensing the position of the gates by reflected sound!

We still have an unsatisfied demand to meet. Canoeing has featured in the local "Talking Newspaper", which has lengthened the queue. Some only do the basic course, relish the experience and retire from the scheme. Others get hooked.

The Thames trip looks like becoming a hardy annual.'

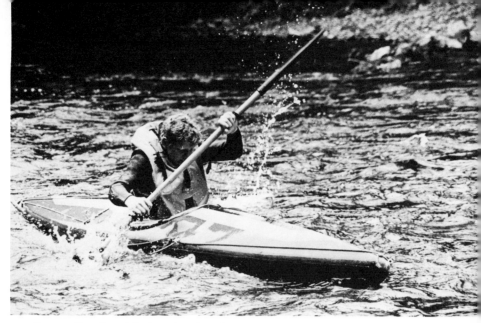

George Scanlin, a blind student from Ysgol Penybont blind school, paddles up the rapids at Symonds Yat.

Anthony Brown, also blind, after a capsize at Symonds Yat.

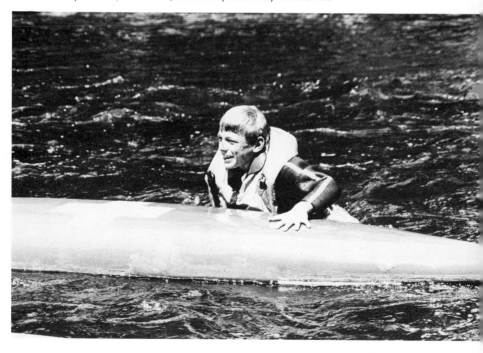

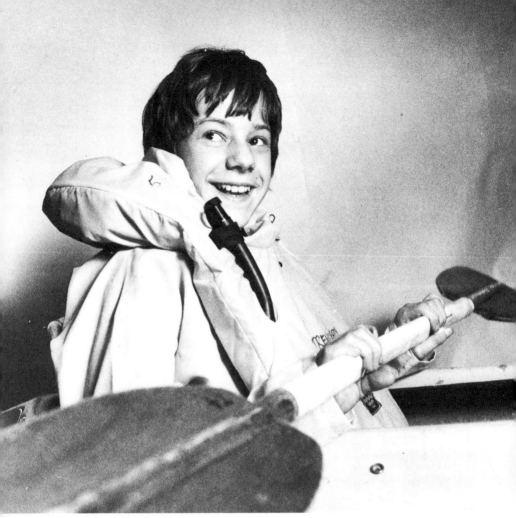

Ian Brewster.

DISABLED? WHO? ME?

Ron Moore is the Regional Canoeing Officer for the counties of Devon and Cornwall and has been working with a disabled group in Plymouth. Recently he was asked to arrange a demonstration at the Canoe Exhibition at the Crystal Palace National Recreation Centre. What follows are extracts from his account of how that demonstration went.

> 'Preparing a display by disabled canoeists presents ethical as well as practical problems. In order to illustrate the various physical handicaps that had been overcome or accepted by our students, we had to reverse

our normal way of behaving by drawing attention to them. When we invited someone to join our display team we asked if we could talk freely to the public about their disability, and in all cases we received their permission to be frank. This was a helpful exercise, as we are so accustomed to underplaying the handicaps that we sometimes lose sight of them.

We asked three leading canoeists to give practical help and it was good experience to rub shoulders with the "great". Our first team member was Darren Evans, 14 years old, who has no strength at all in his legs, although he can walk if he wears calipers. These are cumbersome so he usually leaves them off and comes in his wheelchair instead. His great trick is walking on his hands, which he can do for long distances.

Peter Tucker, 15 years old, was next to appear. He walked briskly along the side of the pool and illustrated extremely well that not all disabled people are easily recognised, since he looks perfectly fit and well. Indeed he is. But Pete was a spina bifida baby and wears a urine tube and bag at all times. He knows he is minimally handicapped compared with other spina bifidas, and both he and Darren have entered several open marathon races, and won some.

Dave Mann is older. He is blind, and works as a telephonist for a Plymouth Bank. In our first display Dave had to walk along two sides of the pool before plunging in and swimming to his boat, and as there were so many obstacles in his way his arm was taken by a helper along this walk. In the discussion afterwards I said that it would be more spectacular if he walked alone to the point where he dived in. So he was pointed in the right direction and given a little push. He always walks at top speed, whatever is in the way, and his nose has scars to prove it. On this occasion he'd taken about six steps, veered too much to the left and fell in. In less time than it takes to say it, he was out again, and walking, just as fast as before but towards me. The rest of his performance, including an Eskimo rescue with Derek, was up to his usual high standard.

All of these canoeists have entered the Devizes to Westminster race this year, with Darren and Pete paddling a K2 in the Junior event. Dave, with a sighted partner, paddled a touring double in the Senior race.

Next to enter was Ross Brewer, another 14-year-old. Ross has general muscular weakness and particular problems with his wrists, which are bent unnaturally inwards. This makes holding a paddle especially difficult. He demonstrated that relatively simple means can overcome apparently big problems by showing everyone his lightweight paddle, made from 1-inch dowel and plywood. He had been very frightened of capsizing, and this was partly because he just didn't have the strength in his hands to pull off an ordinary elasticated spray-deck. Now he has a velcro deck and can paddle in wild water, but if he capsizes his spray-deck pulls off easily. Ross demonstrated a capsize after showing how he can perform high braces, being pulled sideways by ropes tied to the bow and stern of his canoe.

Ian Brewster uses forearm crutches and performs prodigious feats of teetering balance when he climbs into the minibus on them. Each time he goes canoeing he has to change his urine bag, which fits onto an iliac loop protruding from the side of his abdomen. The most notable thing about him is that he's always prepared to go canoeing, never wants to be carried anywhere, makes his own bed and prepares his own complicated drip tubes and night bottle. He did a great job capsizing a Caranoe and showing that even without the use of legs it is possible to be rescued in deep water.

Our final participant was Martin Fuller who has lost the use of his legs and can get out of his wheelchair only with great difficulty. He joined our display team to help us show that seriously disabled people can still canoe, with the proper amount of help and the right equipment. Martin was lifted into a Caranoe by two strong men and towed away by Derek Hutchinson.

We have taken Martin on long expeditions this way, and he's explored Plymouth Sound and the surrounding rivers with a tow on the long arduous stretches and paddling himself on the more interesting parts. We've found the Caranoe an ideal boat for those whose balance is not good enough to keep upright in an ordinary canoe. We have spray-decks for them, and they go on long sea trips, grade 2 white water or small surf.

The display ended with a raft of all students and instructors, with as many as possible standing. As Darren wasn't wearing his calipers he stood on his hands.'

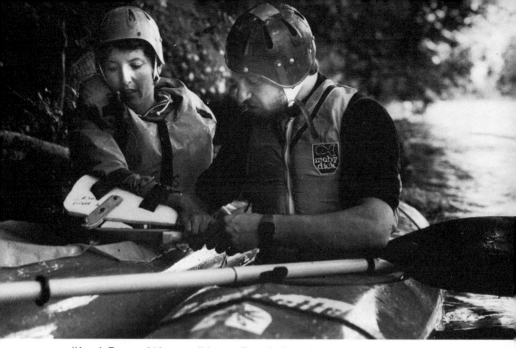

'Kayak France 82': expedition on French rivers by disabled students of the Spastics Society Churchtown Field Studies Centre:
Paul Vander Moden explaining the use of his one-arm paddling device to Elizabeth Hugon, disabled through polio.

Mike Riches using the one-armed paddling device.

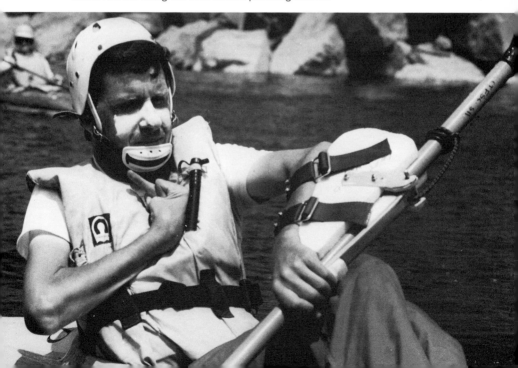

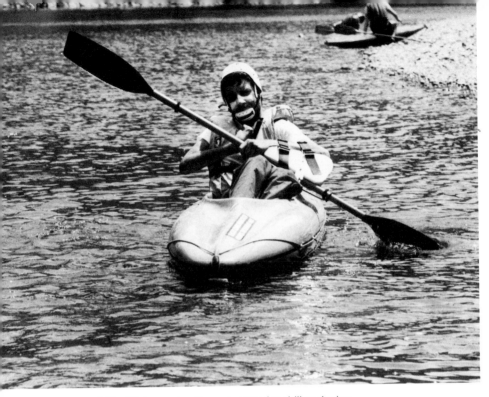

Mike Riches using the one-armed paddling device.

Sue Wiley (both arm and leg disabilities) with instructor John Walker negotiating a stretch of rapids on the Ariège.

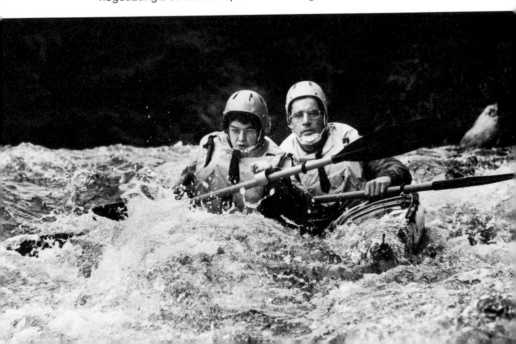

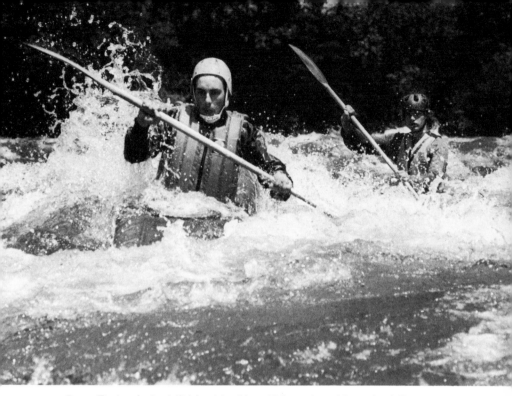

Peter Tucker (spina bifida) guides himself through rapids on the Ariège, followed by instructor Pierre Dabour.

7. Rowing

At first sight the sport of rowing would not appear to offer much opportunity for disabled people to take part. It demands considerable qualities of endurance and muscular strength. Long distance training, weight training and speed interval training are important features of an oarsman's preparation. His purpose is to build up stamina and the ability to maintain a high output of energy over a long period, as well as quick bursts when demanded. But rowing, like most other sports, can be enjoyed in non-competitive ways, or the nature of the competitive element can be adapted to take into account the varied physical abilities of those who are taking part. And provided the disability can be compensated by modifications or the choice of a particular design of boat, the chance to compete in a sport where strength, endurance and tenacity as well as technique are important has proved a rewarding challenge to some disabled oarsmen. The installation of fixed seats, for example, has enabled people with disabilities of the lower limbs to row successfully, since the use of the legs has been reduced.

There are two distinct methods of propulsion: rowing, in which each person handles one oar, and sculling, in which two oars, known as 'sculls', are used. One or the other might suit a disabled person best, depending on the nature of his handicap.

PHYSICAL REQUIREMENTS

Safety on the water is the first and essential requirement. As in canoeing, the important thing is not the distance which can be swum, but confidence in the water should a capsize occur or the boat become swamped. And once again what should be assessed is the ability to cope in cold water under the conditions in which rowing takes place. There should always be close supervision of any crew which has a disabled person among its members.

Deaf people can compete on equal terms with others in rowing. Good teaching using visual demonstration is all that is required. Blind people can also learn to row, and with a sighted cox there is no reason why they should not compete in normal regattas. Their often highly developed senses of hearing, balance and touch can prove to be assets in this sport. The Worcester

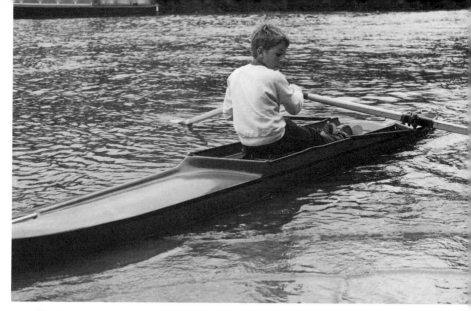

Rowing training at the Worcester College for the Blind:
Ian Sharpe after his first outing in Playboat.

After a successful second session.

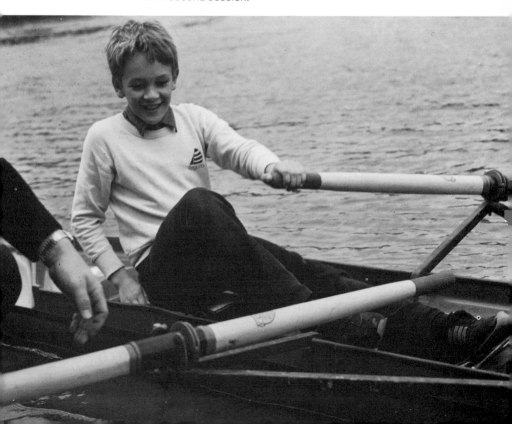

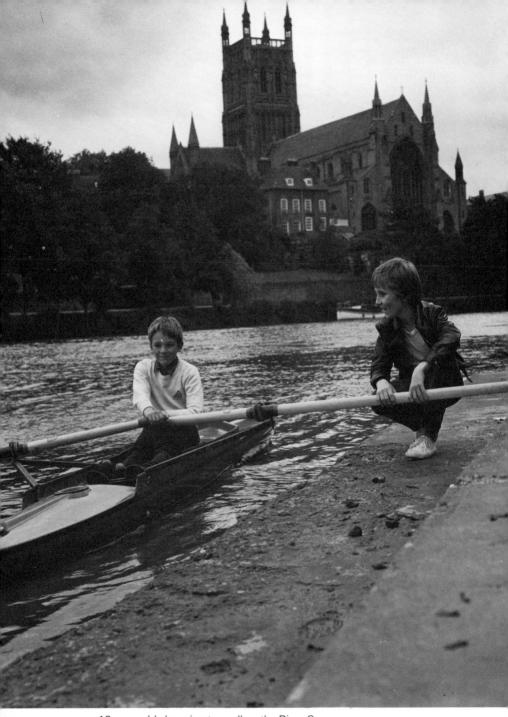

12-year-olds learning to scull on the River Severn.

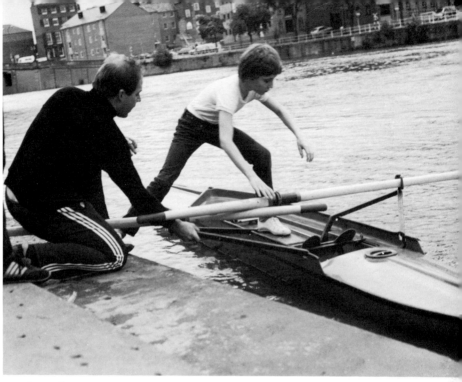

Jason Spencer going afloat for his first outing.

Junior pair.

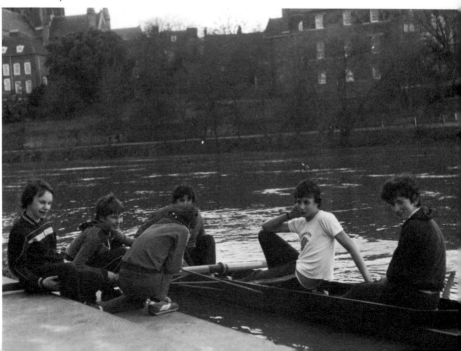

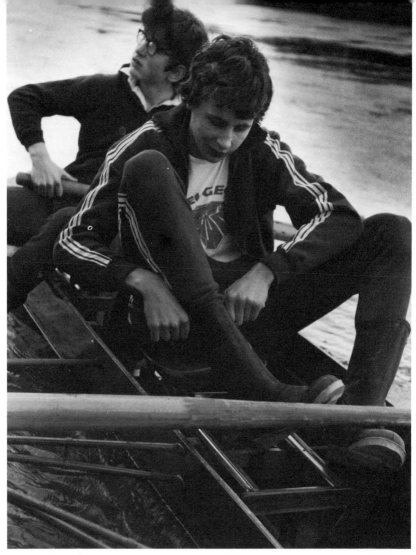

Junior pair.

College for the Blind, for example, regularly turns out crews in all coxed boat classes.

A disabled person with leg amputation below the knee can row quite successfully on a sliding seat. The Henley Royal Regatta has seen at least one oarsman with this disability competing in the pairs event. Modifications to fix the seats have also enabled people without legs to row.

There are now a number of disabled coxes who find their disability does not prevent them from taking part in the sport on equal terms with others.

The essential attributes for a good cox are lightness for racing purposes (50 kilograms or 110 pounds for men, and 40 kilograms or 90 pounds for women and juniors), mental alertness, good eyesight and judgement, steadiness and balance, and deftness in manipulating the rudder lines. The coxswain of the gold-winning U.S.A. eight at the 1974 World Rowing Championship in Switzerland was a severely handicapped person. John Willis and Derek Ward-Thompson have distinguished themselves as coxes in University rowing in England, and both have told how they came to take up the sport in accounts which are given below.

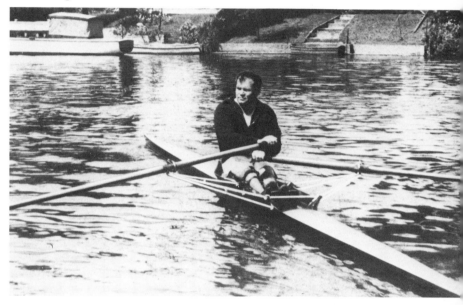

A legless oarsman sculling on the Thames.

A disabled oarswoman prepares to go afloat in a coxed pair.

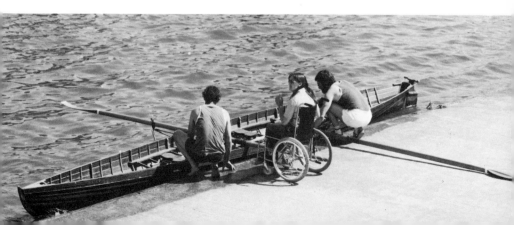

EQUIPMENT

Boats vary from training and touring craft of a more stable nature to highly sensitive and light racing boats. Some racing is still done in fixed-seat boats, particularly in the Thames Valley where it is known as 'skiffing'. In this type of rowing the legs are less important than when sliding seats are used. A recent innovation has been the Playboat, developed by a Nottingham boat manufacturer. (See Appendix 4, p.250.) This is a short but wide sculling boat of plastic construction. It has exceptional stability which allows the basic skills to be learned in safety. Although originally designed to give youngsters immediate return and satisfaction from their first outing, it has also proved to be well suited for introducing disabled people to rowing.

Rowing tanks and bank tubs, if available, can also be used so that disabled people can learn the early stages and techniques of rowing in safety. The former are usually indoors on land, and so the teaching conditions are particularly good for beginners. The latter are fixed to the bank of a river.

Techniques of teaching and rowing will, of course, vary according to the extent and type of disability. Provided the trainee is able to put the blade in the water and apply even a small amount of pressure, a propulsive effect can be obtained and the boat moved through the water. Sometimes it will be easier to propel the boat by pushing the oars away from the body rather than by the traditional method of pulling.

SAFETY

There are traditional safety precautions which are well known and accepted in the sport of rowing. Where disabled oarsmen are involved, however, it is essential to make a thorough assessment both of the limitations imposed by the disability and of the conditions in which the sport is to be practised. The organiser or instructor must be confident that he is not placing the disabled oarsman in situations where his disability can entail avoidable or unacceptable danger. He will not try to remove all risk — risk is an element in most sports — but he must try to foresee problems which may arise, and ensure he has taken precautions which will reduce the hazards to acceptable levels.

Awareness of the nature of the person's disability is important. The following check list is a guide to other areas that require careful attention:

- Stability of the boat
- Buoyancy
- Whether life-lines or lifejackets are to be used

- The water on which rowing is contemplated: still — flowing — tidal — inland or sea
- Should there be an instructor in every boat — in a separate boat — or in a safety boat?
- How many students should the instructor be responsible for?
- What are the problems of embarkation and disembarkation?
- What are the arrangements for first aid and resuscitation?
- Is there a code to cover all emergencies?

'A CHALLENGING AND DEMANDING SPORT'

The following account of how a disabled Cambridge University student coxed a College boat to victory appeared in a recent edition of the Amateur Rowing Association journal *Club News*.

'*Last term John Willis coxed a college boat to victory to chalk up his first win on the river since he took up rowing as a freshman almost a year ago.*

What made that success notable was not so much the race, a short sprint up the Long Reach, nor even the efforts of the crew of the Trinity Hall 2nd Eight. It was a personal triumph for the 20-year-old under-graduate in a battle against a handicap he has fought since birth. For John Willis has two stumps instead of legs and his arms taper to a sudden halt just about where his elbows should be. By winning the "Emma Dashes" up the Cam he made his own unique contribution to the college boat club's most successful term and has put himself in line for the cox's seat in the 1st Eight.

"Somebody as a joke suggested I should start coxing as I was so light," he said. "I went down to the boathouse to try to steer a four and didn't hit the bank — so they put me in a novice boat and I have been on the river every term since."

The boatman rigged up a leather harness attached to the rudder strings so John can steer his boat simply by swinging his shoulders. As he has a more robust build than the average lightweight cox he finds he sits more firmly in the stern and is not liable to be thrown as the boat jolts forward. But the job has other more personal satisfactions. "This is the first time in my life that I have been able to compete on an equal basis, which is why I enjoy it. If I take a corner badly then people can criticise it but not because of my disability," he said.

John, who comes from Upton Cheney near Bristol, was born disabled.

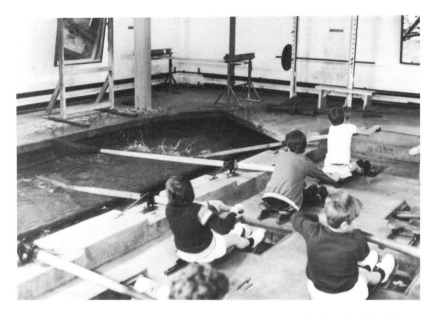

Pupils of Worcester College for the Blind training in the Hereford Rowing Club indoor tank.

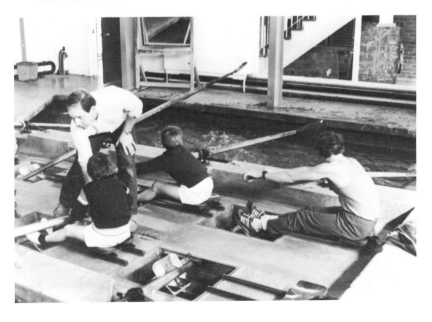

He wore artificial long legs until the age of six but now prefers his specially constructed boots because they enable him to climb stairs. And since he left the company of other disabled children at an early age he has tried to lead as normal a life as possible. He walks short distances within college and to law lectures, though his rowing colleagues push him in a wheelchair to the boathouse, and a rota of friends help him to get out of bed and dressed every day. Despite this he is a very keen supporter of the university rugby and soccer teams and runs the college croquet club. It is the only other active sport in which he can actually take part, although he also learned to swim at school and is captain of one of the college chess teams.

When he finishes his studies in eighteen months, John expects to go to law school to train as a solicitor. "When you get up at six in the morning and everything on the river goes well, it is a really fabulous feeling of togetherness," he said.'

Derek Ward-Thompson is another disabled student who was born with arms little longer than an inch. He reads physics at Christ Church, Oxford, but became interested in rowing at a very early age, when he saw photographs of his father coxing and rowing when he was younger. He decided then that he would like to cox.

'When I started at Durham School, rowing was one of the sports which was on offer, so I put my name down to become cox. I coxed several school crews with varying degrees of success, until in my last two years I coxed the 1st Eight. When I went to Oxford University the competition for places was much tougher. In my first year I reached the last twelve out of forty coxes who entered for trials. In my second year I finished third, only narrowly missing the place of cox of Isis, the Oxford 2nd crew.

Over the years I have learnt the easiest way to alter a boat's rudder lines. Usually two pieces of string are all that is needed. I have always enjoyed coxing. Especially when in the summer there is the routine round of regattas. Four afternoons a week of training, then on a Friday the boat is loaded onto the trailer ready for each Saturday's regatta, where win, lose or draw, everyone enjoys themselves.

Being a successful cox is more than just sitting in the back of a boat shouting. It involves knowing something of the water on which one is racing. It involves steering a fast-moving boat across often tricky water, using only a small rudder, from the start of a race to the finish in the

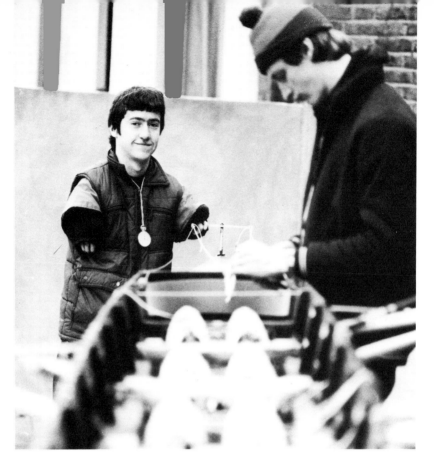

Derek Ward-Thompson makes adjustments to the rudder lines.

Coxing a four on the river.

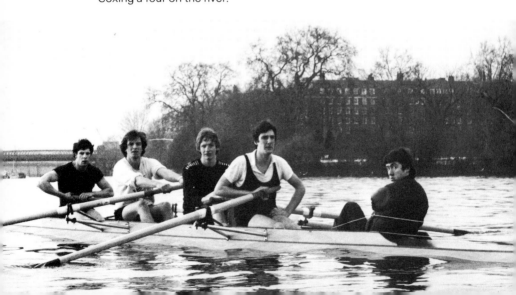

shortest possible time, which is seldom the shortest possible distance. It also involves coaching eight oarsmen in order to bring the best out of them, which naturally requires a thorough knowledge of the technical side of rowing.

I find coxing a very challenging and demanding sport in which, no matter how often I have been out in a boat, I still find something new.'

Mike Downs is an accomplished oarsman though he is a spastic. Only his legs are affected. Mike has a strong, well developed upper body. His walking is somewhat cumbersome, but this does not prevent him from carrying boats. He does not have an oarsman's powerful legs, but he rows in eights, in fours and in single sculling craft.

Mike discovered rowing quite accidentally when he visited a contact at the local rowing club to borrow a book on car maintenance. He was so attracted by what he saw that some of the members invited him to come and have a try.

They put Mike up at the bow and told him to follow what they did. He was very frightened at first, then got used to it. He has even fallen in when making inevitable mistakes.

Mike does not use any modifications. He believes that integrated activity is the only way to do it. He thinks that all disabled oarsmen should know how to swim but not necessarily be strong swimmers. It is the training he likes, along with the fellowship of being a member of a good club on equal terms with others.

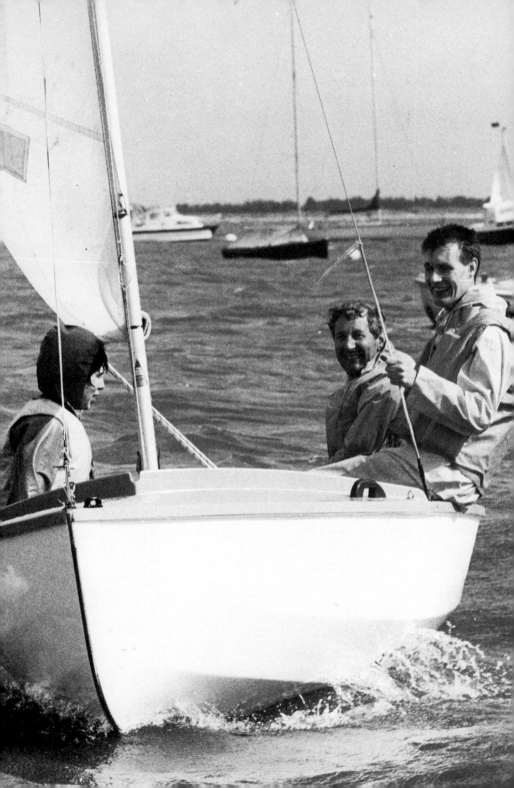

8. Sailing

Boating in its various forms, whether for fun or as a serious sport, attracts an increasing number of participants of all ages. The thrill and challenge of pitting skill and knowledge against the elements, in all their moods, cannot easily be surpassed. With proper supervision and safety precautions the sport can be a source of relaxation, pleasure and discovery to a great many disabled people.

There are already a number who have shown that their handicap need be no barrier to the higher levels of the sport. Ken Roberts, for example, although confined to a wheelchair, has qualified as a Royal Yachting Association Coach, teaching both able-bodied and disabled people to sail. He also runs safety boat courses at his local outdoor pursuits centre.

Diane Pattinson was already a keen sailor when she became a paraplegic as a result of a serious accident, but she returned to the sport. *'It just seemed natural to take it up again.'* She is now married and has less time for sailing. *'But,'* she says, *'sailing offered freedom and fresh air. The fact that I was on a par with the next boat pushed the whole idea of being disabled into the background. It became unimportant.'*

Diane Pattinson busy during winter maintenance.

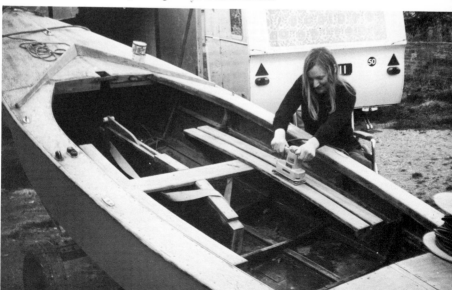

Arthur Slater, minus a leg, has for many years been one of Britain's most successful ocean sailing skippers, and, indeed, is a former 'Yachtsman of the Year'.

'When my left leg was amputated at the thigh as a result of a crash in the Monte Carlo Rally, my world of work, motor racing, sailing, fishing, swimming, water skiing and, would you believe, dancing, was completely shattered. Or so I thought.

Sitting in a hospital bed contemplating my position I decided that the only thing to do was to try and ignore the disability, and to sail my Dragon type yacht became my first goal. Motor racing, unfortunately, was out, but within weeks I was deriving immeasurable pleasure from many of the sports which I had enjoyed previously.

For the amputee taking up a water sport, one of the greatest fears, probably, is the risk of "phantom limb" or nervous pain as a result of getting wet. I can only say that I have been half-drowned, experienced extreme hot and cold and even been lost at sea — soaked and starving — for four days in a Force 9 gale, without having any discomfort in the amputation area. Yet sitting at home in a draught has resulted in real problems.

In the 1974 Cowes Week regatta, I borrowed a 42-foot yacht from a friend and entered the Nab Tower Race, a distance of approximately 30 miles. With one exception we were a disabled crew with only five legs out of a possible fourteen. Some of the crew had very little sailing experience and much of the equipment was quite new to them. Nevertheless we finished eighth out of sixty-eight starters. Their reaction to competition and their ability to participate on equal terms with the able-bodied was a joy to see.'

Individuals like these, who refuse to be deterred by their handicap, will say that anyone who is determined enough can extend his horizons. It is encouraging to see the number of youngsters who, with the aid of experienced sailors, are following their example.

EQUIPMENT

At times a sailing dinghy appears to be the wettest, coldest and most uncomfortable vehicle imaginable. Strangely enough this is part of the attraction of sailing. But it is important to wear proper clothing: a properly fitted wet suit when sailing dinghies, water and windproof clothing for larger boats, and plenty of padding.

It would take many pages to list the variety of craft available. Boats fall

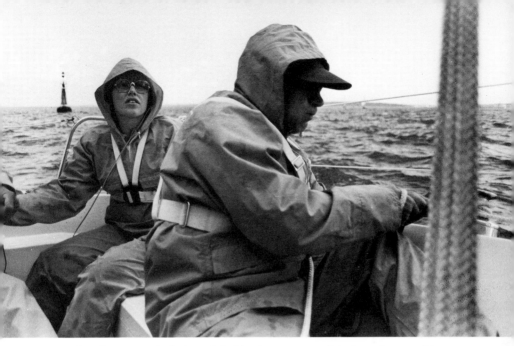

Good water and windproof clothing in a gusty spell during a Seamanship Foundation course for the visually handicapped. The helmsman is wired up for the audio compass.

broadly into the classes of sailing dinghies; yachts (usually over 6 metres (20 feet) in length) powered by sail and engine; and motor cruisers, which are motor-powered only. There is also the dayboat class with fixed keel, popular for day sailing. Dayboats are more stable than dinghies and should be particularly suited to handicapped people.

The type of boat will obviously determine the type of sailing the participant will do. It is common sense for the beginner to crew in a boat before buying one, to ensure that sailing is a sport he will like. He will also be able to decide on the form of sailing he prefers. Many people start with small boats and then progress to bigger craft. Others often become attached to their first boats, and continue to sail them happily for many years.

When special modifications have to be made to boats or equipment, they must allow the disabled person to fall away from the boat in the event of a capsize. These additional fittings (e.g. sliding seats, shortened tillers and extra grab handles) can assist trainees with certain handicaps to achieve better control. Under no circumstances should a person be restrained or strapped in. In general, disabled trainees are encouraged to sail ordinary boats under ordinary conditions. Those who wear artificial limbs should remember that salt water and mild steel do not get on well together! So an old one should be worn or a way found of keeping vulnerable parts protected.

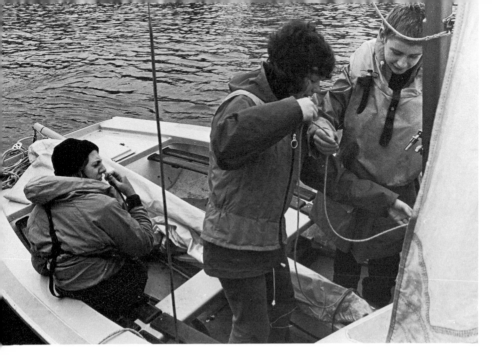

A disabled youngster shown how to rig a Wayfarer during a course at Ravens Ait on the Thames.

He takes the helm under instruction.

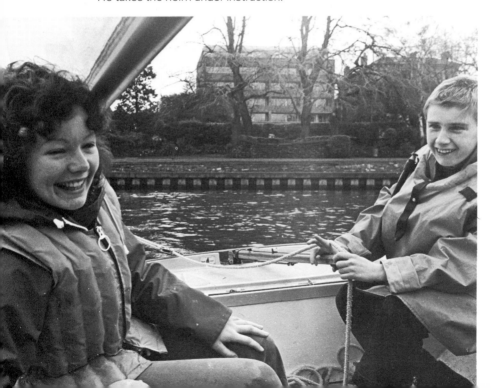

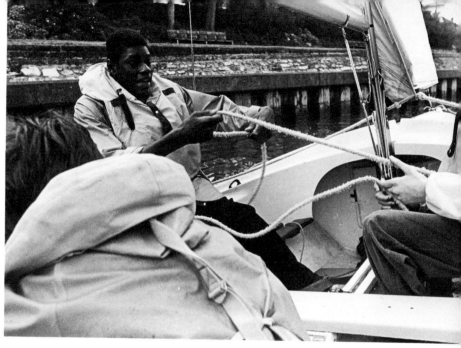

A polio-handicapped boy learns how to handle the jib sheets during a Ravens Ait course.

The tiller is often a problem for the handicapped helmsman.

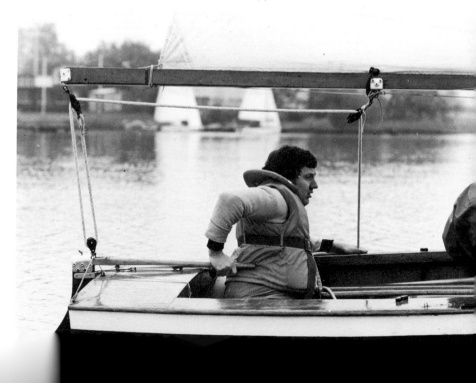

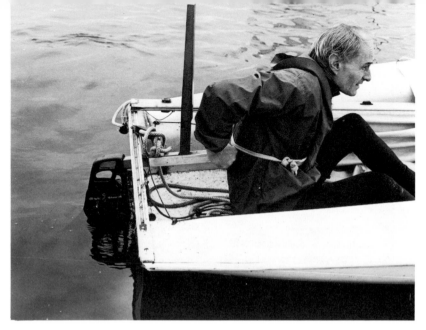

A shortened and hinged tiller gives more room for manoeuvre.

PHYSICAL REQUIREMENTS

The two major problems handicapped people find in sailing are getting into the boat and, once aboard, moving about the craft. The larger and more stable the boat, the easier it can be to get aboard and the less need there is to move about to keep it balanced.

In the main, however, it is necessary to be able to move quickly when sailing small boats, and the ability to use hands and arms is an obvious requirement. 'To what degree?' is the question most frequently asked by disabled people interested in taking up sailing. This will depend on the type of craft and how active a role in crewing the boat the disabled person wishes to take.

Some will be able to aim at helming the boat and taking command of it. Others will be able to crew, while some will be passengers.

Both mental aptitude and physical ability must be considered in deciding whether a handicapped person is able to sail small boats. If there is minimal or no arm control, then unfortunately controlling or helming are impossible, and crew duties also. If a person so handicapped still wishes to sail, however, he can be taken out by a competent crew and still experience the pleasure of being afloat in a small boat. Great care should be exercised when taking mentally handicapped people in small boats. They should always be accompanied by someone who is not only an expert sailor but also understands their range of ability. Special caution is necessary with those suffering from epilepsy. Reference should be made to the section dealing with this handicap on p.17.

The ability to swim, however limited, is essential. A swimmer is less likely to panic in the event of a capsize than a non-swimmer. It also follows that a recognised lifejacket or buoyancy aid, preferably fitted with a crotch strap, should be worn at all times when afloat.

For those handicapped people who have arm control and co-ordination, sailing a fast dinghy can be a stimulating challenge and experience. Inability to move quickly about the boat need not be a big handicap. It is possible to obtain mechanically operated sliding seats to assist movement from one side of the boat to the other. However, independently controlled seats are still not sufficiently controlled and tested.

Don Riddle, a polio victim, is helped aboard after capsize drill.

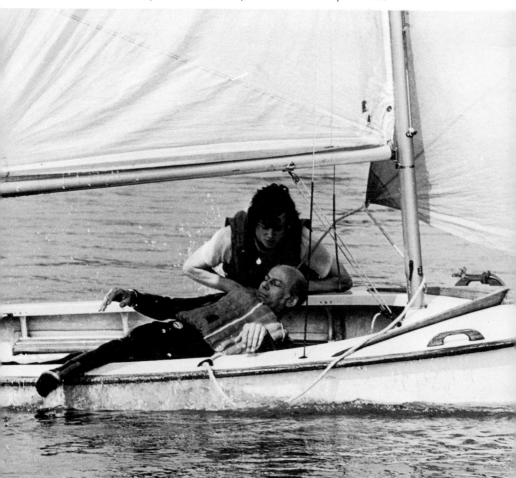

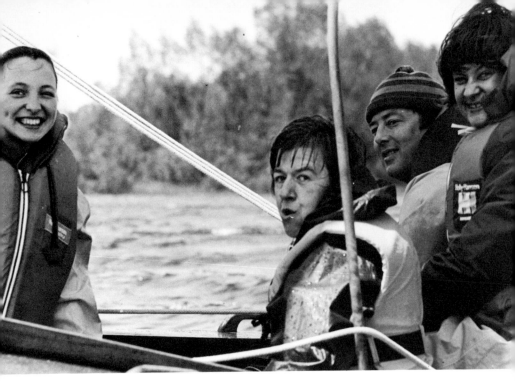

Disabled sailors under instruction during a course at the Naseby Sailing Club.

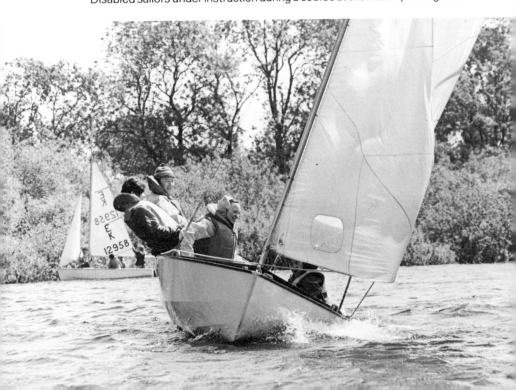

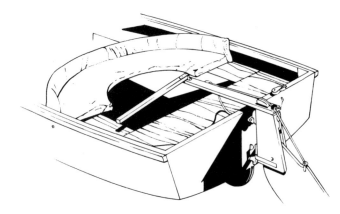

The Curtis Seat, designed to enable a paraplegic helmsman to slide easily from one side of the dinghy to the other.

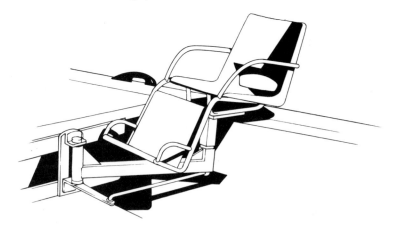

The helmsman's swivel seat, allowing easy movement on changing tack.

INTRODUCTION

In introducing handicapped people to sailing, the main aim should be to ensure that safety measures are observed. For this reason it might be better for the disabled beginner to attend one of the 'Sailing for the Disabled' events, such as a club open day, so his aptitude and physical ability can be assessed. It will also give him a chance to find out if he likes sailing. Once he has been introduced to sailing the disabled sailor is in a much better position to approach his local club.

It is at club level that organisations such as the Sports Council, the Royal Yachting Association, the Spastics Society and many other interested bodies can be of greatest service to the handicapped. These organisations can pave the way to full club membership, and therefore to total integration. Club members will have to appreciate the difficulties which face the disabled sailor while he is still on land. Afloat he may have other problems but often he will be as capable as anyone. He will need help in getting the boat rigged and into the water, and then in getting into the boat. When coming ashore and recovering the boat the disabled sailor will also need the help of his club mates.

In small sailing dinghies a ratio of one handicapped person to one able-bodied crew should be strictly applied. In large dinghies, two disabled and two able-bodied people has proved a good combination. There are many examples of handicapped helms taking part in club dinghy racing with an able-bodied crew.

Vaughan Davies, a paraplegic as a result of a motor accident, at the helm of a GP14 getting ready to sail on Lake Windermere.

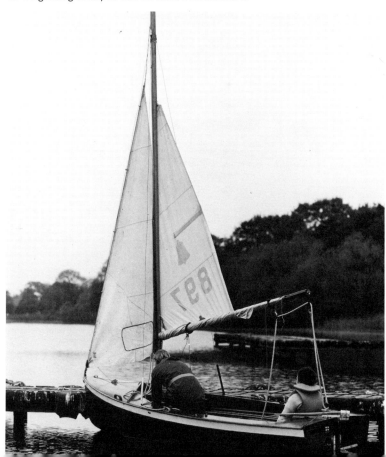

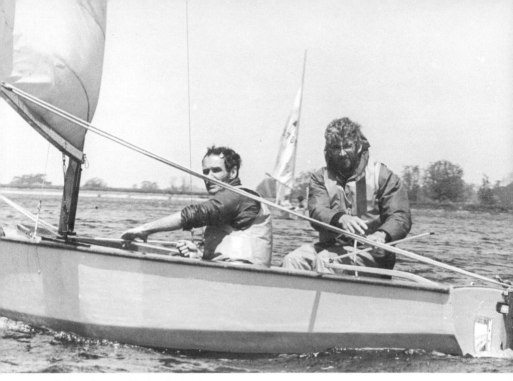

Going about: able-bodied helmsman and blind crew.

A theory class in session at Ravens Ait.

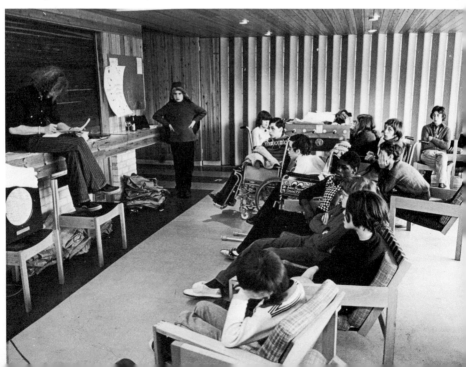

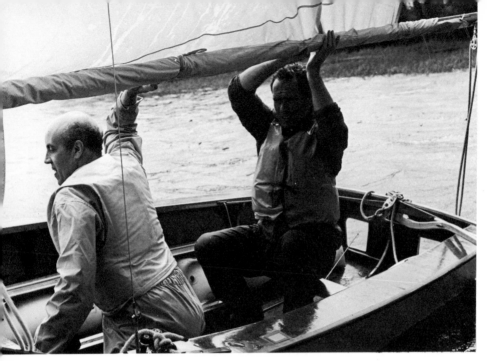

Lowering the well-reefed mainsail at the end of the sail on a gusty day.
Blind helmsman and able-bodied crew.

Help is needed to get the disabled person aboard.

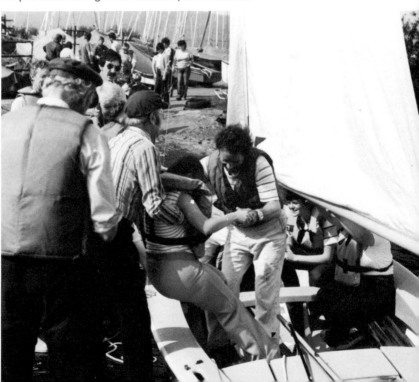

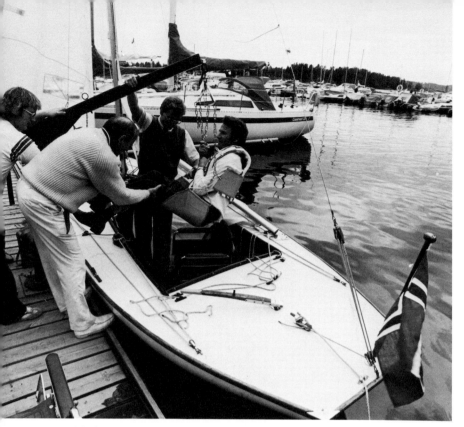

A hoist makes it easier. Per Blix, a Norwegian paralysed from multiple sclerosis, is lowered into a swivel chair on transverse rails from which he is able to helm the boat.

Bob Bond, the Royal Yachting Association's former Training Manager, writes:

'Ideally, instruction for disabled people is carried out on an individual basis within a club. However, a number of special courses have been arranged for the handicapped including those confined to wheelchairs and the blind. Information collected from such courses is available to course organisers.

Once again, the R.Y.A. favours a policy of integration as being most beneficial to the disabled person. Such a policy will ensure that those organising courses will normally have only one or two disabled persons on each course, and the bulk of the work of helping the disabled will thus be carried out by other course members.

Some excellent examples of integration have already occurred in

*many parts of the country, and show that development along these lines
is succeeding.*

*As already explained, sailing is defined as an 'at risk' sport – so
everyone must be able to look after himself in cold water wearing a
lifejacket or buoyancy aid (see section on 'Lifejackets and Buoyancy
Aids', p.207). The minimum requirement, as already stressed, is the
ability to sit up in a boat unaided, one good arm for pulling ropes and
operating other simple controls, alertness and quick reactions.*

*Blind people have a particular aptitude for dinghy sailing, because of
their increased perception and concentration. Deaf people also make
successful sailors.*

*Finally, sailing need not be expensive. Many owners·do not have
regular crews and are happy to welcome fellow sailors in this role.
Personal protective clothing and lifejackets will be needed, and a club
subscription. It is often possible to purchase a second-hand dinghy at a
modest price to start off with.'*

Malcolm Fisher reading a Braille chart of the Solent.

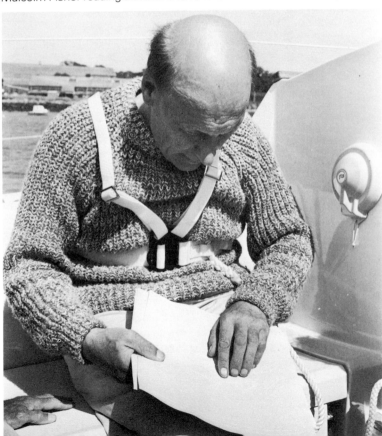

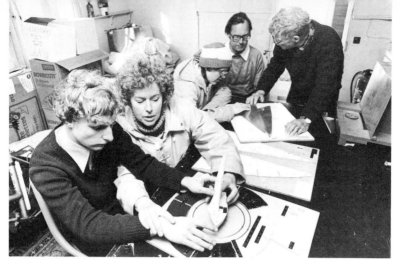

John Sugden, Heather Taylor and Peter Eckersley being taught the theory of sailing using tactile training aids.

The U.S. Hobie-Cat. A disabled crew returning from a sail on a lake in Colorado.

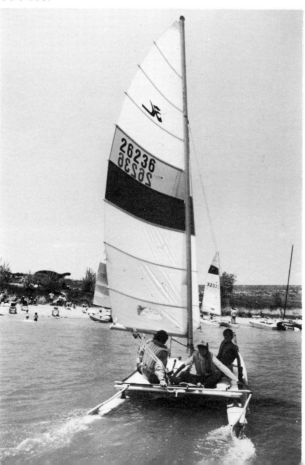

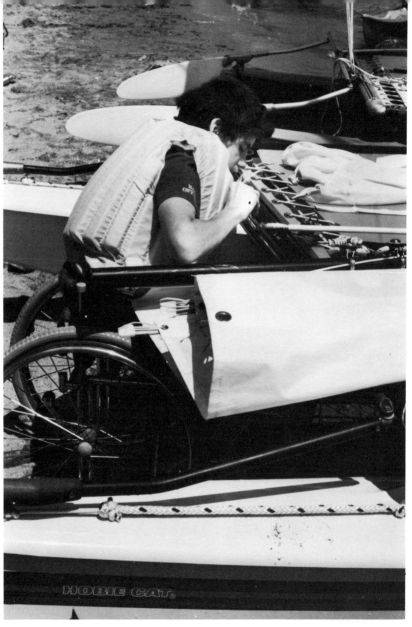

Disabled crew making adjustments to the tiller of his Hobie-Cat.

Facing: Peter Eckersley preparing to hoist the foresail. Seamanship Foundation course for the visually handicapped.

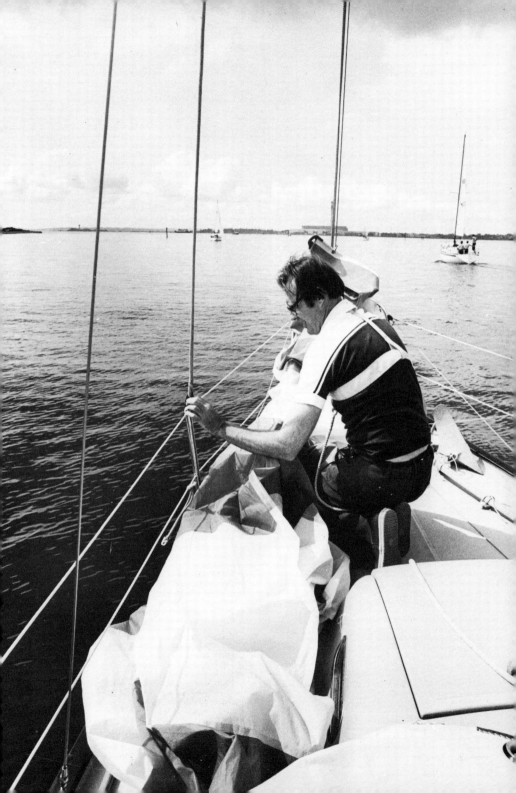

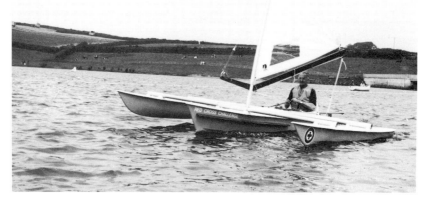

The Seamanship Foundation Trimaran *Challenger*, specially designed to be sailed single-handed by paraplegic sailors.

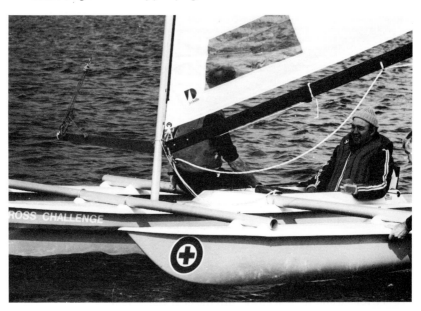

9. Coastal Cruising

Disabled people who are interested in sailing but are worried about going out in dayboats or small dinghies may feel more confident in bigger craft. If the weather is reasonable, day sailing on cruisers can be quite relaxing and attractive because it combines sailing with living on board and visiting different harbours and anchorages.

Seamanship skills

Taking a cruiser out to sea requires various seamanship skills, many of which can be learned by disabled crew members in order to play an active part in running the ship. Navigation, weather forecasts, radio communication, cooking and look-out duties are all important jobs for which physical strength and agility are not the first essentials. Taking the tiller, changing sails, and other types of deck work need more mobility and balance.

Limiting the numbers

The number of people on a cruiser depends on its size and how many berths it has. Small craft between 5 and 8 metres (17 – 25 feet) long can usually accommodate from two to three persons, while medium-size 9-metre (30-foot) cruisers may sleep four or five. On ordinary coastal passages it would be impracticable to have more than one disabled person in the crew, but on some of the larger vessels used by maritime youth training organisations this number could be increased.

Modifications

Structural alterations to provide easier access above and below decks are undesirable, because they could reduce a vessel's seaworthiness. Additional fittings such as grab handles and steadying rails can make it easier to move about, and non-ambulant crew members might find sliding or bridging boards useful for horizontal transfers. Wheelchairs and walking frames, including the narrowest models, cannot be used on board, and aids of this nature should be folded and stowed away until the next visit ashore.

Space on board

For those who have difficulty in walking, the risk of falling obviously increases with the greater horizontal and vertical distances to be negotiated on bigger boats. On the other hand, the limited space available on small cruisers can cause discomfort and stress to the inexperienced beginner, and the unsettling effect of a short sea is felt earlier. Regardless of the size of the vessel, people who cannot walk often find that the greatest problem is the access to the toilet compartment. This should be one of the first points considered when planning a cruise which includes handicapped people. Disabled sailors may be able to suggest ways of overcoming the problems, but usually some independence has to be sacrificed, unfortunately in a situation where it is most prized.

At present, disabled sailors must content themselves with whatever facilities are available on production vessels. The size offering the best compromise in space and safety is in the region of 9 metres (30 feet), with six berths and a clear entrance between cockpit and cabin, usually a drop of 1.5 metres (5 feet). Wheel steering and roller reefing are standard boat fittings which enable people with limited reach and mobility to take a greater part in handling the boat. Other helpful features such as a helming seat can be introduced if desired.

Getting on board

Unlike their enthusiastic helpers, most disabled people regard getting on and off the vessel as a somewhat risky and unpleasant experience largely out of their control. The process of being hoisted in a sling or bosun's chair from a jetty or small boat onto a cruiser should be accepted by leg disabled people as the safest and least troublesome way of going on board. A competent crew can easily boom a person over the side of a cruiser and this is the method which should be used wherever possible.

Day sailing

Day sailing and cruising in coastal waters offer an adventurous and rewarding opportunity for integrated activities involving disabled and able-bodied youngsters. They are certain to be more popular among the handicapped as more and more people spend their leisure time in outdoor pursuits. There should, of course, always be experienced and competent cruising sailors among the able-bodied members of the crew.

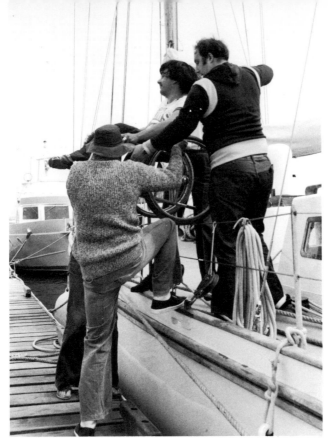

This is hazardous for the disabled person and the helpers alike. A boom or hoist should be used wherever possible.

Ken Roberts giving instruction on knots in a quiet period in the marina.

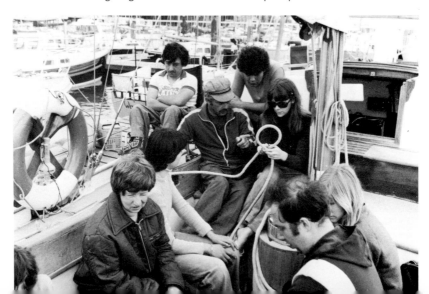

HOW TO MAKE A START

Cruising vessels can cost about the same as a small house or bungalow, and their upkeep is almost as expensive. Because of this, most people charter or hire a cruiser when they want to go offshore cruising, and all they need to take is their food, sleeping bags and spare clothing. A list of reliable cruiser hire firms may be obtained from the Yacht Charter Association (see Appendix 4, p.250). Charter fees will depend on the size of boat, the season, and whether it is accompanied by a professional skipper. Newcomers are often asked for a reference.

Individuals or very small groups wishing for experience in coastal cruising may be able to enrol for a yacht cruising course with one of the R.Y.A. recognised sailing schools. Many of them offer an interesting and active holiday with instruction provided if required.

A P.H.A.B. group at the end of an Ocean Youth Club cruise to Cherbourg and Guernsey.

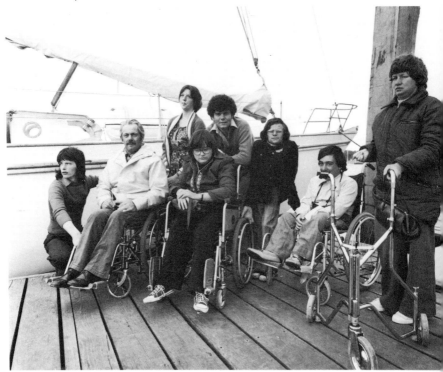

Equipment

The following equipment has been found useful when there are disabled people among the crew.

- *Multi-purpose harness* for deck work and for hoisting on and off.
- *Monkey rope* for access up and down companion-way below decks.
- *Folding stool* for transferring inside cabin, and getting to places where there are no seats.
- *Star mooring hook* on telescopic pole for tying up.

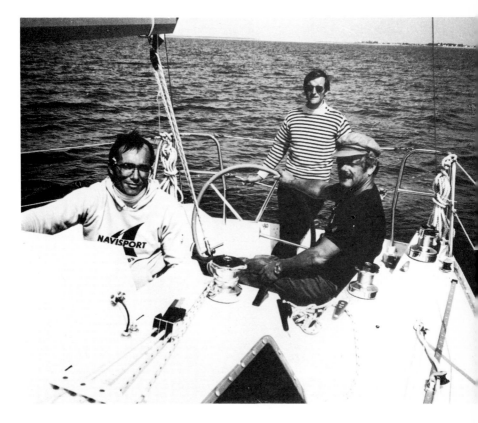

L'Ecureuil, the second of two 29-foot sea-going cruisers launched in 1982 in France for use by disabled yachtsmen. Conceived by Alain Floch, himself a paraplegic, and operated by Navisport, Nantes, they are designed to overcome the problems and discomforts which he experienced in sailing standard craft. Paraplegic skipper and crew.

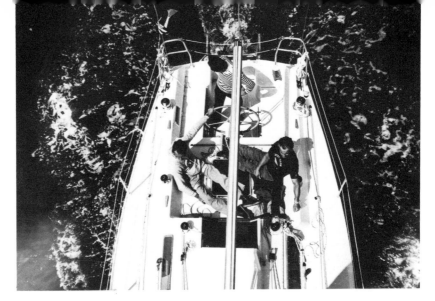

Roomy cockpit with padded seating and controls brought aft.

Seat which can be cranked up from cabin to cockpit.

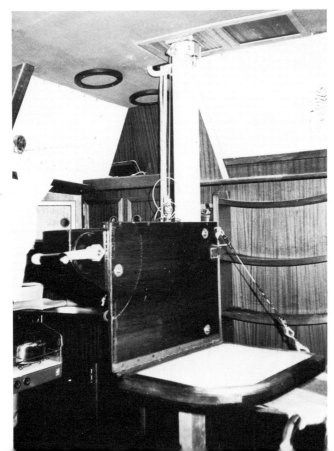

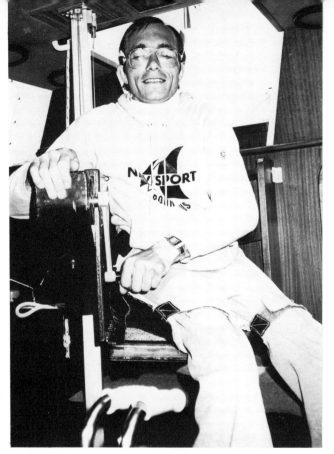

Paraplegic skipper cranks himself up.

Twin rudders in the up position.

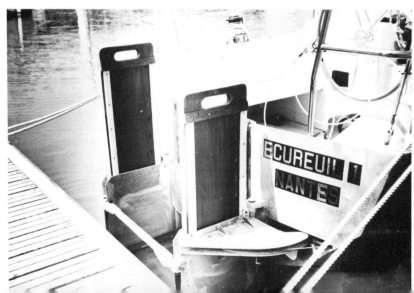

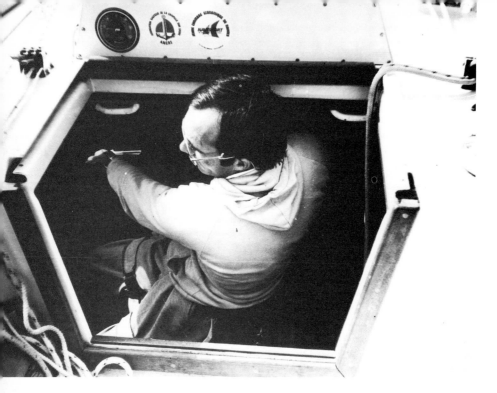

Emerging through the hatch. Note the protective padding.

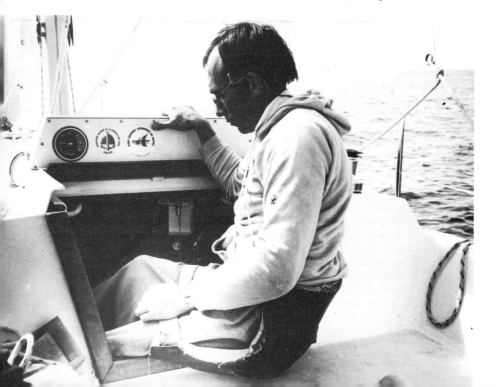

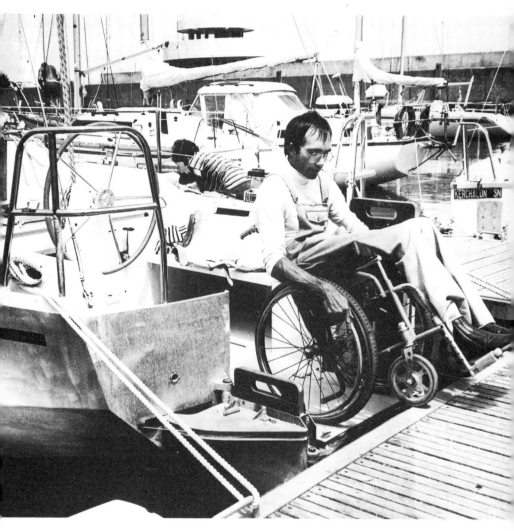

Disembarking using the stern 'gang plank'.

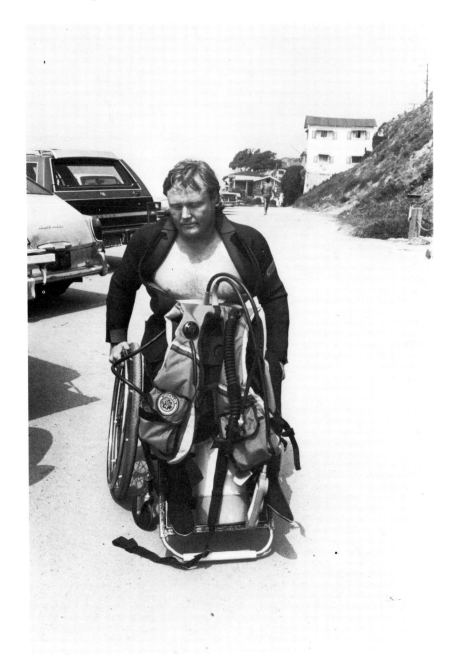

10. Sub-Aqua

In spite of the strict necessity for medical fitness in diving, it has long been apparent that a person with a quite serious injury, one leg amputated above the knee for example, can, other things being equal, become a competent diver.

The British Sub-Aqua Club has explored the possibilities for disabled diving for some years. Its policy is to encourage branches, at the discretion of the branch diving officer, to accept disabled members for diving training wherever possible.

In view of the risk entailed, particularly outdoors where circumstances often make supervision difficult, it may seem foolhardy to encourage people who have already suffered severe injury to take part. However, the risk need be no higher than with able-bodied people. The essential art is to learn how to maintain the risk within acceptable limits by modifying the techniques and restricting the tasks attempted.

Disabled people can be safe divers and active branch members, provided that the proper medical precautions and checks are made first. There is no reason why a disabled diver should be a 'passenger' in the branch.

PHYSICAL REQUIREMENTS

At this point it should be made clear what is meant by a seriously disabled person, and what degree of self-sufficiency is aimed at in training. In the context of diving, the amputation of one leg is not serious, because many people can swim well with one leg. There are problems in walking about wearing the equipment, but they are not medical or physiological problems, nor peculiar to diving.

The absence of a hand or arm is more serious, since a diver frequently has to adjust his equipment while underwater. However, the difficulty is one which can be overcome, given careful supervision and instruction by a good diving instructor, who must judge the safety of the pupil. There is no special medical problem.

A special danger for paraplegics is that they do not know the position of their legs unless they look at them. This is difficult while wearing mask and scuba, and so there is a risk that their feet or knees will collide with rocks, coral or wreckage. If complete suit covering is worn there is little risk of abrasion or cuts, but in the absence of a suit, extreme care must be maintained.

In view of the particular hazards, diving is not suitable for people suffering from epilepsy, and they should not take part.

TRAINING

It is preferable that severely disabled people should receive initial training at special short courses supervised by doctors and physiotherapists.

Disabled divers should not dive with each other. After receiving initial training, the trainees should join an active diving club or diving school. Training in these organisations is usually carried out on a part-time basis over many weeks or a few months, and this is ideal for the disabled person. By diving regularly with members of the club or school, the disabled diver will acquire a group of friends and fellow-divers who know his capabilities and limitations when diving at sea, and this will provide maximum safety.

Disabled divers should, as far as possible, complete all the established training exercises as laid down by the *Confédération Mondiale des Activités Subaquatiques*, and be granted the appropriate certificates. The C.M.A.S. standards of training should only be reduced or modified to allow for restricted depth and sea conditions, and in respect of life-saving, since the disabled diver can give very little assistance to others.

The disabled diver who acquires sufficient sea experience to become qualified should receive a certificate or log book endorsement stating clearly the limiting conditions within which he may dive safely. He should receive an annual medical check to ensure that it is safe for him to continue diving.

LEVEL OF COMPETENCE

The level of competence which should be achieved is as follows:

- The disabled diver is passed as medically fit to dive so that his companions do not have to worry about him. He can drive himself to the dive site and look after his own diving equipment, but may need assistance getting into a boat, and fitting his scuba gear in the water.
- Once dressed he can swim unaided, dive, adjust his equipment, perform all the normal safety exercises, swim in the company of a buddy diver, monitor the progress of the dive, control his ascent, and swim to the boat on the surface. At the boat he will probably require further assistance to remove his equipment and to get back on board. If he becomes separated from the boat he can inflate his lifejacket and so survive for many hours.

● This level of independence ensures a high degree of safety, and permits the disabled person to join in diving groups of able-bodied people to enjoy underwater observation, photography and natural history, or underwater science and research.

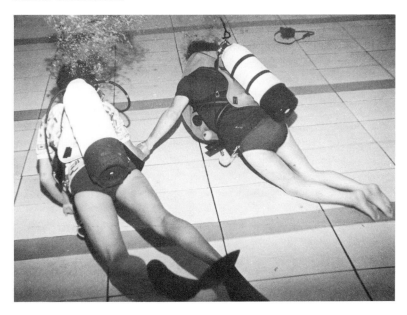

Disabled trainee working with able-bodied 'buddy' in swimming pool. Buddy using flippers to propel both along the bottom.

This paraplegic trainee must develop strong arm stroke for propulsion.

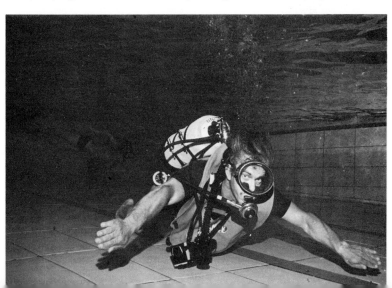

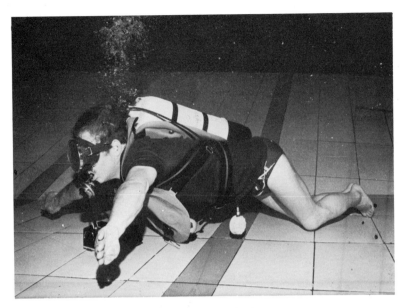

There is a danger of scraping the knees on the bottom.

The disabled trainee learns how to control movement and position in the water by practising forward and backward rolls.

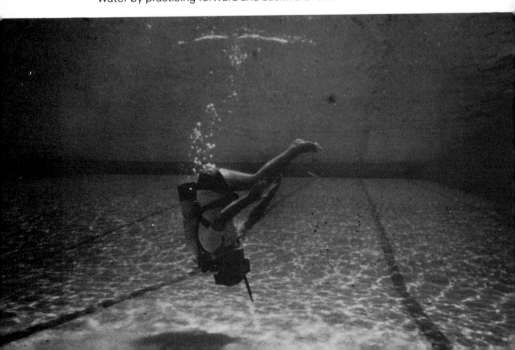

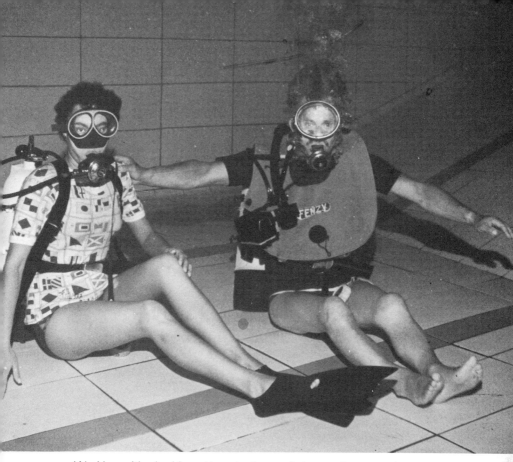

Working with a buddy and learning how to balance when seated.

All divers must learn to breathe from a fellow diver's aqualung system in case they run out of air.

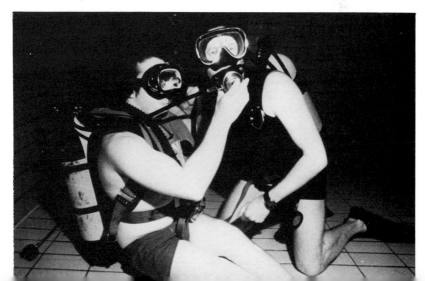

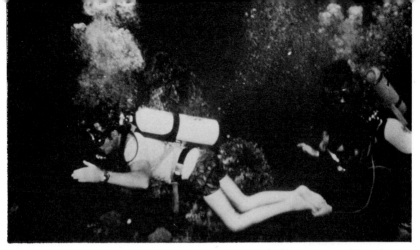

The disabled trainee dives in open water accompanied by two experienced buddies who watch his progress and are ready to assist if necessary.

The disabled trainee holds himself down by draping his weight belt over his knees and removes his facemask. The next step is to replace the mask and clear water from it by an exhalation through the nose.

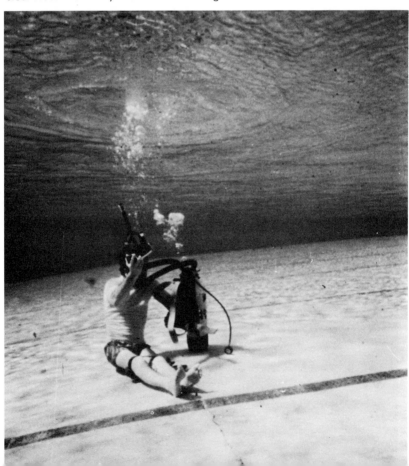

ACCESS TO THE WATER
Access points

The technique of entry varies at different locations. Very broadly these are of three types:

1. shelving beach of sand or gravel
2. steep wall of rock, concrete or stone, such as a jetty, or a wooden catwalk
3. a boat or ship

If the disabled person can walk, then the technique is very similar to that recommended in all competent diving manuals. If the disabled person cannot walk, the technique is modified to allow entry to the water, and to allow the diver to put on his diving equipment.

Shelving beach

For a person who uses crutches, walking across a beach may be very difficult. Equally, a wheelchair tends to sink in. However, in both cases the student can get close to the water with some assistance. Mask and fins should be washed in sea water and freed of sand. If he cannot walk, the student can transfer from the chair to a sitting position on the beach, and then move on his hands through the swash zone into the water until it is 0.3 – 0.6 metres (1 – 2 feet) deep and he can almost float. Then he can put on the mask, and the fins if they are of use. If aqualung gear is being used, a friend should bring out the tanks and weightbelt and help the diver to put them on. The diver should then swim through the waves straight out into deep water, taking care not to scrape his knees on the bottom.

This technique obviously works only in a very calm sea. If the waves are more than 0.3 – 0.6 metres (1 – 2 feet) high, a paraplegic will be rolled over and his skin abraded on the beach. In this case, one or two strong able-bodied friends should carry the diver through the breaking waves until he is floating in unbroken water. There the aqualung equipment can be put on safely, and the dive commenced. The return to the beach must of course be very carefully supervised.

Jetty, dock or catwalk

Diving is often carried out in or near harbours, and entry may be from a steep wall with steps. The situation is very much like a swimming pool with high walls. For snorkelling, the swimmer may be thrown into the water by two friends. This may sound brutal, and should not be done without warning any soft-hearted tourists who may be around. However, if a wheelchair snorkeller puts on mask and snorkel while sitting in the chair, and is picked up by shoulders and ankles, he can be thrown quite safely into the water from a height of several feet. The mask must be held so that it does not get knocked off.

If the dock is too high, friends will have to carry the disabled diver down the steps. Once in the water, aqualung gear can be put on in the normal way. Maximum assistance is obviously needed to get back up again.

Boat or ship

From a rubber inflatable craft, it is a simple matter for a disabled diver to roll over the side into the water. When returning to the boat, the diver removes all his gear in the water so that people on board can pull it back. They then assist the diver on board.

Getting out of the water into a motor launch with hard wooden, metal, or fibreglass edges is one of the trickiest problems for a paraplegic diver. With a vessel of 5 – 10 metres (16 – 33 feet) there will probably be no ladder or davits. The vessel will tilt if a lot of people move to one side but the gunwales will still be high enough to be very awkward. If there is no ladder, the gunwale should be heavily padded with canvas, sacking or blankets. Two men should lift the diver out (after he has taken his aqualung off in the water), and a swimmer should stay in the water, possibly between the disabled diver and the hull of the boat, to ensure that his thighs and legs are not scraped.

If there is a ladder, the disabled diver should take a secure hold on the shoulders of a man in the water, who then walks up the ladder with him. Assistants should catch the disabled diver's legs and help them over the gunwales.

It is unusual to dive direct from a large ship. The divers usually transfer to an inflatable or power launch. If diving is from a yacht or ship with high sides, there will usually be a companion-way. The situation is then very much as when diving from a dock wall. If the diver is strong enough, it may be simplest for him to climb down and up a rope hanging from the davits, or be winched up and down in a crane or on the davits.

Note

A competent disabled diver is safest when he is well away from boats and the shore. When he is near rocks, jetty pilings or the shore, his lack of full mobility becomes a hazard, especially in a rough sea. Entry to and exit from the water requires great care, and plenty of strong assistants. More assistance is needed at this point than when he is actually diving.

SAFETY

Basic rules

The following basic rules for sea diving should be strictly observed by disabled people:

- Obey all usual diving regulations and medical regulations concerning diving.
- Your safety factor is *always* lower than for an able-bodied diver.
- The dive begins when you leave home and ends when you get back home safely.
- Never dive alone.
- Always dive with two able-bodied experienced divers close to you in the water; i.e. within 5 metres (16 feet) or visibility range, whichever is the smaller.
- There must be at least one diver and a boatman in the cover boat.
- Always plan and survey your entry into and exit from the water with the people who will be helping you.
- Ensure that your diving companions know your limitations in terms of diving safety, and general medical care.
- You cannot use your hands to adjust your equipment or carry out work while you are swimming. Avoid situations which require both at once.
- Never dive in a current stronger than you can swim against for a long time.
- Avoid abrasions and cuts from reefs and rocks. Do not touch corals.
- Do not make dives requiring decompression stops.
- Never go under overhangs.
- Never go inside caves or wrecks.
- Never dive at night.
- Never dive in visibility less than 3 metres (10 feet). It is impossible for your companions to stay sufficiently close to you to give rapid help in these conditions.

DEVELOPMENTS IN NORTH AMERICA

Perhaps most progress in introducing disabled people to diving has been made in North America.

Canada

At an International Conference on Underwater Education held in Toronto, Canada, in November 1981 the National Association of Underwater Instructors of Canada (N.A.U.I.) presented a programme and course outline

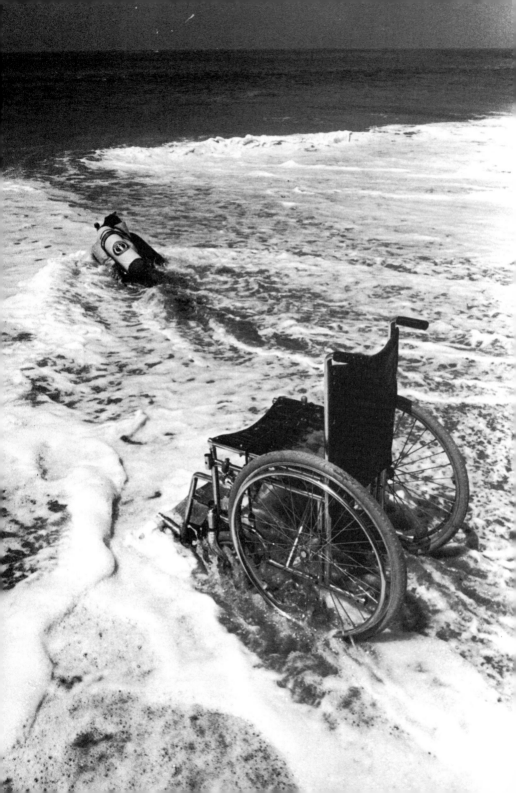

put together by instructors who had been teaching the physically disabled over the previous two years. Emphasis is placed on the partner or 'buddy' system where an able-bodied and disabled diver are teamed together. While the framework of the normal N.A.U.I. course is adopted, alterations to facilitate the teaching of the disabled are described.

The work of the group with handicapped children in the Hospital for Sick Children, Toronto, is chronicled in a film entitled *Free Dive* (see Appendix 4, p.250). This film shows children who are wheelchair-bound, or have difficulty walking on land, becoming free underwater and exploring the environment like any other diver. The youngsters are victims of such handicaps as spina bifida, cerebral palsy and paraplegia. After learning to use masks, snorkels and flippers in the hospital pools, they eventually donned wet suits and swam in open water. By this time they had earned their skin diving certificates. As a culmination, they were invited to the Grand Cayman Island to explore the beauties of the coral reef. *Free Dive* shows a prototype programme for teaching the handicapped to dive, and is an affirmation of their capacity to enjoy a rich and varied experience.

United States of America

The following account appears by courtesy of the Handicapped Scuba Association:

'*Anyone standing at the surf's edge in Laguna Beach, California, one summer day in 1975 would have witnessed a puzzling sight — empty wheelchairs parked upon the sand. Where were the occupants of these abandoned chairs? Set free to explore the ocean's boundless beauty as certified scuba divers. An unusual event? Certainly, but a dramatic and rejuvenating achievement now possible for many highly motivated disabled people.*

Seven years ago, through the efforts of a veterans' service organisation at the University of California, the Handicapped Scuba Association was set up. Classes began in the University swimming pool and then spread to nearby beaches for surf-entry dives and culminated in a spectacular boat trip to Catalina. Today the H.S.A. continues to hold sport diving classes in which the able and disabled are paired together in a 'buddy' system that greatly enhances the experiences of both divers.

In a potentially dangerous situation where each diver must depend upon the other, the able-bodied diver discovers unknown capabilities of the disabled while the latter discovers previously unknown deficiencies of the able. The water minimises the differences between them. Much of

*the limitation experienced on land by a handicapped person is
eliminated once he is in the water.*

    *Apart from its formal class structure the H.S.A. operates as a dive club,
offering refresher courses, co-ordinating recreation beach dives and
scheduling dive boat excursions for its qualified members.'*

And what do the handicapped divers themselves think?
Thirty-five year old Larry, paralysed since childhood:

'*I jumped at the chance. As a disabled person in a wheelchair I had
always assumed that anyone else not in a wheelchair could do any
physical activity better than I could. It was quite an eye-opener that
they could have the same difficulty with tasks that I did. And some
tasks I could do better than men without a disability.'*

Mike, injured in a car accident which left him paraplegic with a lesion so
high that he even lost the use of his stomach muscles:

'*It's tough but it's something that gets us out of our wheelchairs. A lot of
people said we couldn't do it, but we did.'*

Scuba diving was the first physical sport Mike attempted since his injury
in 1967. Now he plays basketball, bowls in two leagues and participates in
wheelchair tennis.

Left: On the Laguna Beach, California. Two members of the Handicapped
Scuba Association make final adjustments before diving.

Right: The H.S.A. have perfected a special technique for entering through
the surf which is a feature of California beaches.

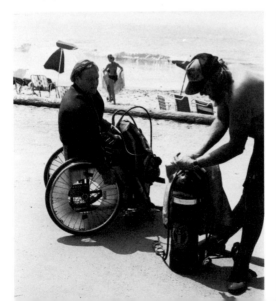
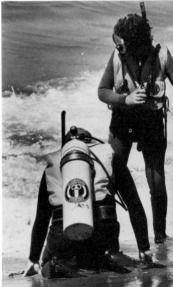

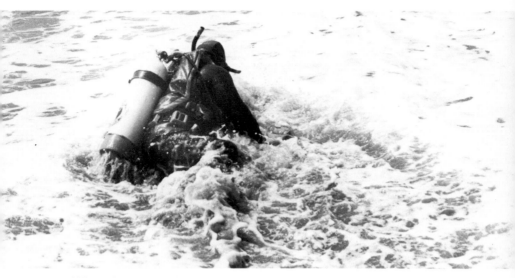

When the water is deep enough for flotation the two divers swim quickly through the surf zone, keeping close together for safety.

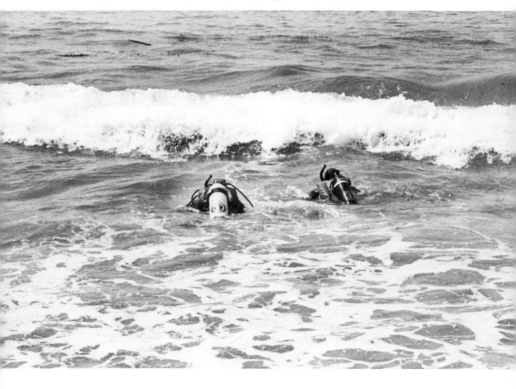

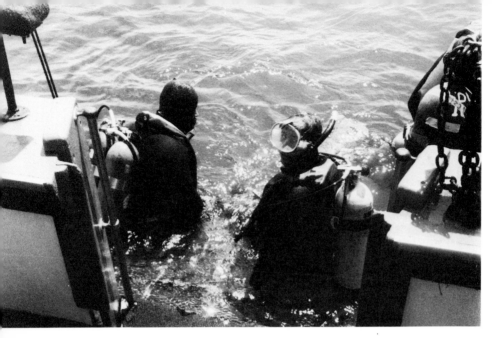

Boat dive. The special swim step at the stern allows easy exit and re-entry for paraplegic as well as able-bodied divers.

A spastic diver returning from a sea dive using the swim step.

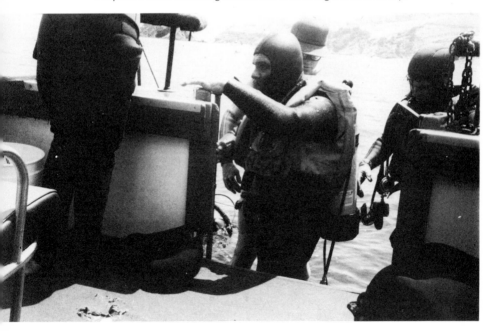

11. Water Skiing

PHYSICAL REQUIREMENTS

Water skiing, although it is no more dangerous than other water sports, is nevertheless demanding in short-term physical effort and involves frequent falls into the water at speed. This unfortunately rules out participation by the more severely disabled. A strong back and three or four limbs in sound condition are the basic physical requirements, although there is at least one water skier with only one arm and one leg. However, he was an experienced water skier prior to his accident.

As with all sports for disabled people, what counts is how keen the person is. Keenness, encouraged by experienced coaches using modern teaching techniques, can allow the basic skills to be learned relatively quickly. In any event a medical adviser should be consulted before water skiing is attempted, if there is any doubt.

It should also be emphasised at the start that in referring to 'disabled people' the blind and the deaf, not only the physically disabled, are most certainly to be included.

The very considerable benefits disabled people can derive from water skiing come partly from the exercise, and the need to maintain a reasonable physical condition to get maximum benefit from time on the water. Even more important, perhaps, is the peculiarly exciting mental satisfaction. Of course it is also beneficial for the handicapped to take part on equal terms with the able-bodied in an adventure sport that still has some glamour attached to it.

As with many of the other sports described in this book, the disabled water skier must have complete confidence and control when left alone in cold water. So long as the motivation is strong, there are no age barriers. Skiing for double amputees and paraplegics (although it is not considered practicable for a person with spinal lesion higher than L1) poses special problems that need to be individually assessed. The use of modified surf boards such as the 'Sitz-ski' and similar sled-like devices is being actively explored. For safety reasons water skiing for the mentally handicapped has not so far been attempted or encouraged in Britain.

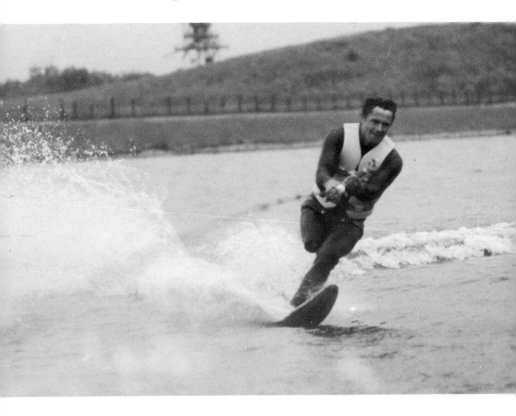

EQUIPMENT

Unless the water is very warm, which is never the case in the British climate, the handicapped beginner should always wear an adequate wet or dry suit and also a lifejacket. The equipment may be borrowed at a club, but the special requirements of limb amputations and paralysed limbs are best met by individually tailored wet suits. All manufacturers will make special suits but it is best to discuss the design with experienced water skiers beforehand. Besides warmth, the wet suit provides important protection for stumps and paralysed limbs. Quite naturally a beginner may be reluctant to purchase equipment until he is sure he is going to enjoy and continue the sport. The 'spare' arms or legs of borrowed suits can always be safely strapped out of the way as a temporary measure. As to skis, they can be borrowed in the first instance from a club or a friend. Normal skis for beginners should be used until experience has been gained as to the most suitable type.

THE BRITISH DISABLED WATER SKI ASSOCIATION (B.D.W.S.A.)

In 1979 the Association was formed as an independent body registered as a charity and having its own constitution and committee. It is affiliated to, and has close links with, the British Water Ski Federation. There are two classes of members: Full Members, who are disabled, and Associate Members, who are not disabled but who are interested in helping the disabled. Associate Members are very welcome, as help is always needed, but the Constitution provides that at least half the members, both of the Association and the Committee, shall be Full Members.

In 1977, David Nations, O.B.E., who had been so instrumental in putting Britain on the water-skiing map, was appointed President of the World Water Ski Union Group II Commission for disabled water skiers. He asked Tony Edge to become the first Chairman of the British Disabled Water Ski Association. Tony originally water skied on two legs in 1937 in the south of France, lost a leg in the R.A.F. during the war, and has been water skiing on one leg since 1959.

The first aim of the Association is to encourage disabled people to take up the sport and make them, the water ski clubs, and the general public aware of the possibilities it affords. A training programme is in hand, both for the disabled and for the coaches to train them. The first residential course was held at Lake Windermere in June 1979, in which four people each with only one leg, one with only one arm and three totally blind people were successfully coached. A second even more successful course was held in 1980 at the Holme Pierrepont National Water Sports Centre.

Once a disabled person has mastered the techniques of getting up and skiing, he should be quite capable of skiing behind his own boat, joining a water ski club or skiing on holiday. In fact he can enjoy the sport in every way with his able-bodied friends.

INSTRUCTION
General requirements

Every effort should be made to compensate a person's disability by making conditions as easy as possible. Calm or sheltered water conditions should be chosen wherever possible. The quicker a disabled skier is on the plane, the less the strain, therefore a powerful boat is essential. This should be at least 100hp for a single skier and with three up on a wide bar, 200–250hp. A disabled skier is more than normally dependent on the skill of the driver. It is therefore absolutely essential that the driver be fully experienced.

Any instructor must be a fully competent skier. He should be a coach trained on a B.D.W.S.A. course, and conversant with the latest training techniques and equipment.

Wide tow-bar

The B.D.W.S.A. has found that the most satisfactory way of teaching both the blind and those who have lost the use of a limb is with a wide tow-bar. An instructor is positioned on either side of the student. Each instructor places one hand inside that of the student on the bar so that support is given under his armpits on both sides. Regardless of disability, the student can then be lifted into a skiing position by the instructors. With this method the emphasis is first on learning to ski on the water after being helped up. Then, as balance and skill are developed, the student learns the more difficult feat of getting up into the skiing position unaided. Initially a one-piece tow-bar with adequate buoyancy floats should be used. It is attached at four points equally along its length to a single heavy-gauge tow-rope. It should be about 2 metres (6½ feet) long.

A development of the one-piece tow-bar is the 'Edge Triple Bar' which, when put together, is of the same dimensions, but consists of three finely engineered metal tubes which telescope together for starting. These can be slid apart while skiing into three separate handles with three individual ropes, enabling the instructors to separate completely and smoothly from the student and leave him to ski solo. Such equipment is the most successful so far developed to effect the transition from skiing with instructors to solo skiing.

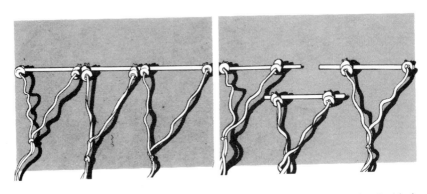

The Edge Triple Bar. The three metal tubes slide apart to enable the disabled skier to ski solo.

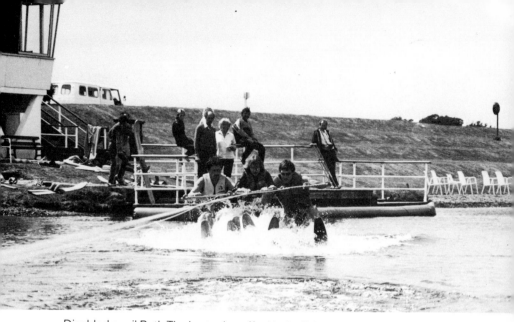

Disabled pupil Ruth Tipple starting off with the Edge Triple Bar and a helper on each side.

Note the position of the inside hands of the helpers, enabling them to support the disabled skier under the armpits.

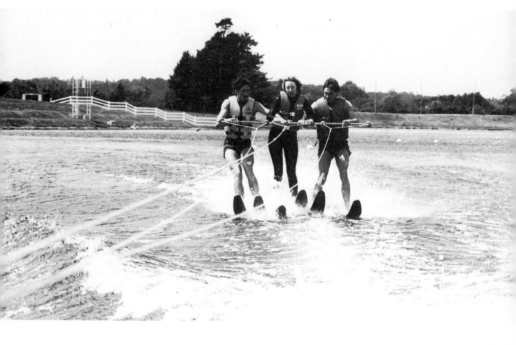

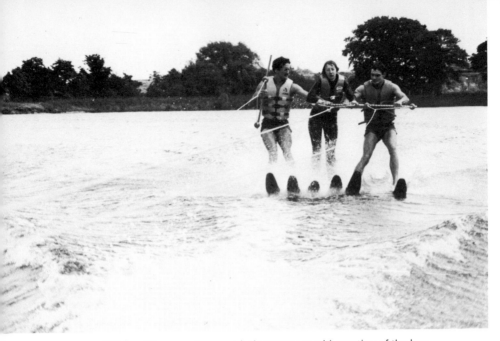

While still supporting, one helper removes his portion of the bar.

Continued support with the bar now completely separated.

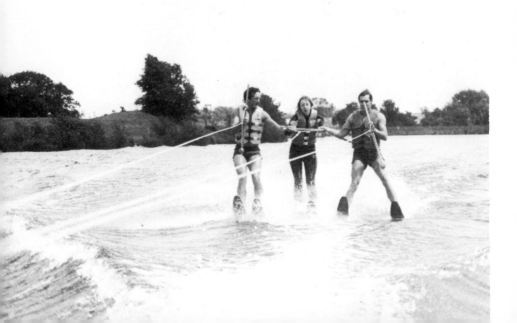

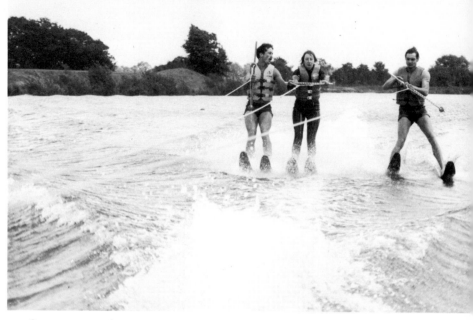

One support only, and much encouragement.

The thrill of skiing solo for the first time!

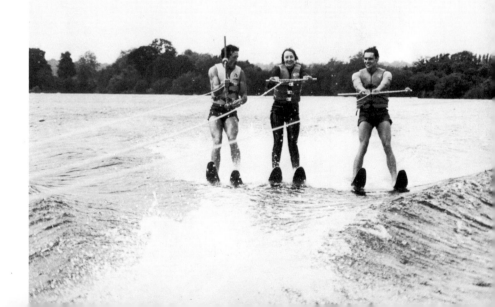

Instructor skiing alongside in tandem, with separate handles and ropes.

This is the natural progression from the wide bar. Two tow-lines are used. The instructor holds his own handle with one hand and firmly grips the upper arm of the student in the water with the other. He helps his student out of the water into the skiing position. The instructor can then talk to, guide and reassure the student, all the time teaching him as he goes along. Once the student is steady, the instructor can relax his grip and allow him to ski independently while still giving him instruction. This method allows smooth and easy transition from complete reliance on the instructor for getting up, to getting up independently and skiing solo.

Getting up unaided takes some mastering, particularly for the leg amputee. Alfred Millard (left) uses the double bar with Robin Nichols.

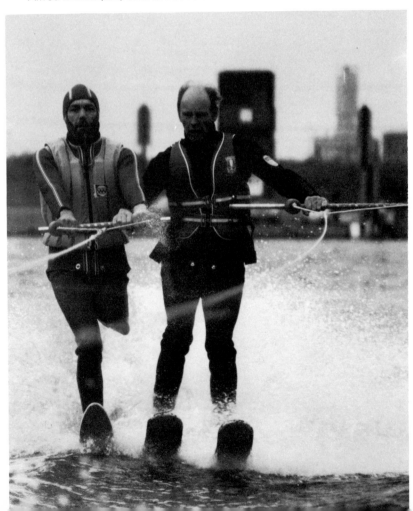

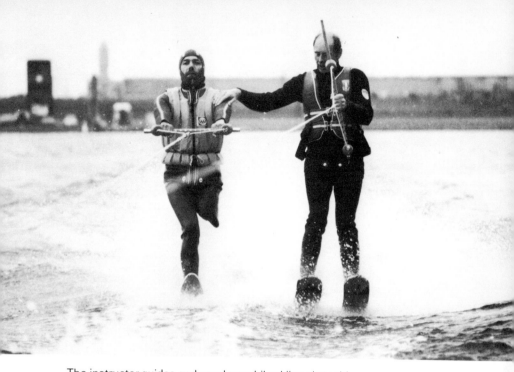

The instructor guides and coaches while skiing alongside.

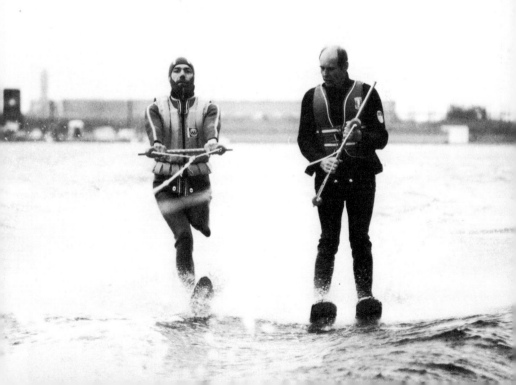

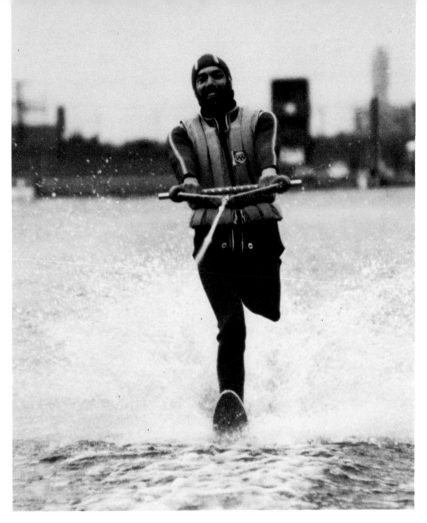

The final independent stage.

Ski booms

Ski booms from the boat are commonly used in water ski clubs for instructing barefoot skiing. The B.D.W.S.A. has found these booms can be useful, mainly at a later stage, in training disabled skiers, depending very much on how they are fitted, the type of boat to which they are fitted, the extent of the bow-wave etc. A fully experienced driver is absolutely essential and it must be appreciated that the close proximity of the boat, with the noise of the engine and the thrash of the propeller, may at first be unnerving to a blind person or someone who has already lost one limb.

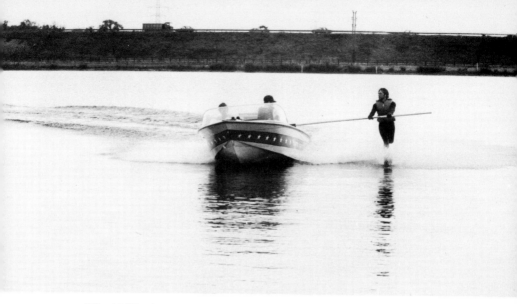

Alfred Millard uses the ski boom for more advanced practice.

PARTICULAR DISABILITIES

Each person's disability is unique to him, and brings its own particular problems which he will have found his individual ways of overcoming. Anyone instructing disabled people must realise this and appreciate that a method which may be successful with one pupil will not necessarily be so effective with others, even though they may have the same disability. There are also, of course, considerable variations in the degree of disability arising from the same cause. Each case requires individual attention. Nevertheless, there are certain groups of disabilities which have problems in common to a greater or lesser degree.

The blind

This appears to be by far the largest group of disabled people for whom there are properly organised camps and training schemes, mainly in the U.S.A. and Canada. The initial training methods explained earlier have been used with success. With an instructor alongside there is no difficulty in giving training instructions or keeping the pupil informed of water conditions, wash, turning etc. For the blind, the B.D.W.S.A. recommends solo water skiing only for fully experienced skiers in properly controlled conditions with an established code of sound signals. Trick skiing, slalom wake crossing, even barefooting and jumping, are all well within the capacity of an experienced blind water skier.

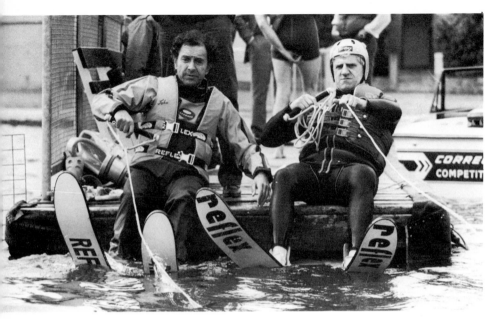

Blind skier Gerald Price (right) getting ready for jumping practice with instructor Peter Felix.

Left: Being guided into the correct path of approach to the jump.
Right: A good position leaving the top of the jump.

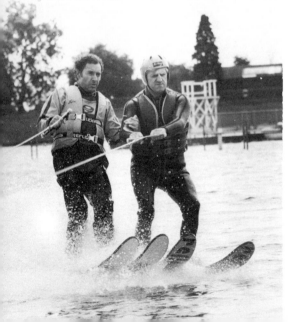

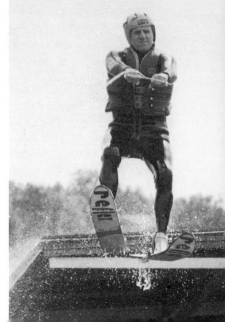

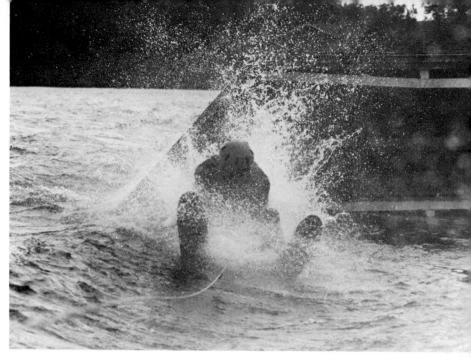

And a successful landing in a haze of spray.

But not too successful this time!

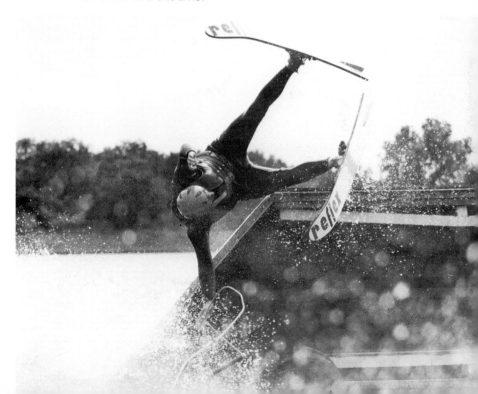

The deaf

For the deaf there are hardly any basic problems in learning to ski other than establishing positively understood visual signals between the driver and the skier before starting. Normal techniques can be learned from readily available books. A special club has been formed for deaf water skiers. (See Appendix 4, p.250.)

Loss of, or loss of use of, an arm

Those with paralysis or amputation of an arm can achieve near normal skiing ability by use of a 'Delgar' sling. A modified handle with a cap which fits over its end is attached by a sling to a harness round the shoulder. The pull on the handle is thus shared between the good hand and the body via the sling and the harness. Release from the device is instantaneous when the good hand releases the handle.

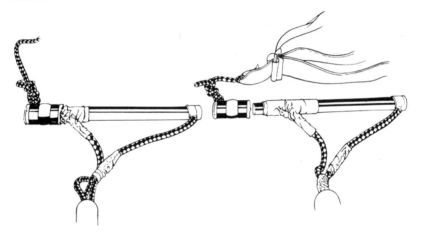

The Delgar Sling and handle. The cap is detached immediately the handle is released.

Lower limb amputees, or loss of use of or damage to a lower limb

People suffering from disabilities of this kind can be considered in two groups:

1. those with injuries or paralysis to the foot, or with amputations below the knee and an artificial below-knee leg which can be waterproofed and thus used for skiing;
2. those who can only use one sound leg for skiing.

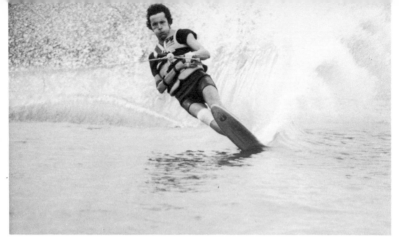

Despite a paralysed right arm and restricted movement of the right leg, Mark Addison slalom skis with the Delgar Sling.

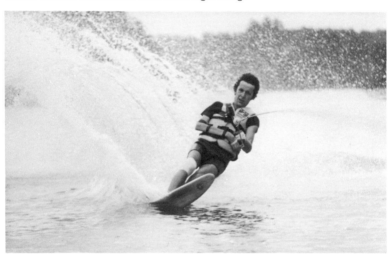

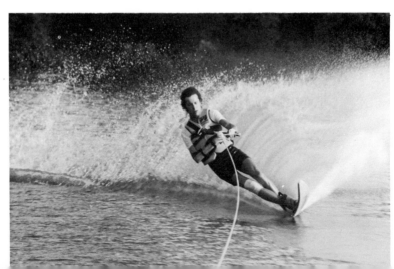

The first group, depending on the amount of control and leverage they have on the damaged or artificial leg, can be taught to get up and ski on their own relatively easily. From that stage they can graduate to mono-skiing, using the damaged or artificial leg in the rear binding. There is even a disabled Canadian skier who uses his artificial leg, very successfully, for jumping.

It is the second group which offers by far the greatest challenge both for the pupil and the instructors; in effect it means learning to mono-ski right from the start on one leg only. Using modern techniques with the triple bar, a complete novice can be skiing on his own after only three days. However, there is still the problem of getting up unaided. The next stage is in tandem, with the instructor skiing alongside. So far no-one has produced an aid to bridge the gap between being helped up by the instructor in tandem and getting up unaided. Getting the knack is purely a question of practice and hard slog, but success is well worthwhile when it is finally achieved.

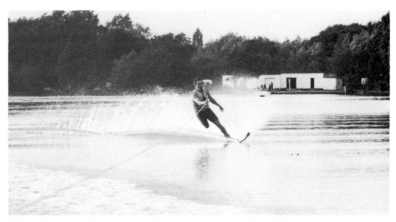

Mike Hammond lost his right leg in a motor accident. He is now a fully qualified snow and water ski instructor.

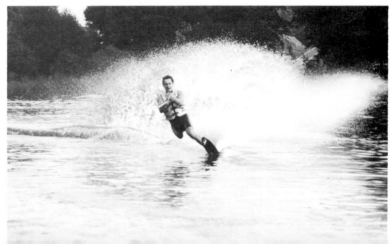

SAFETY

Disabled people who take up water skiing obviously have an adventurous nature. Nevertheless it is most important that anyone already suffering from a disability should not be exposed to further unnecessary risks for the sake of his sport.

As the result of experience, sometimes rather painfully gained, the B.D.W.S.A. has drawn up a special code of practice. This can be obtained free on application to the Association. (See Appendix 4, p.250.) Anyone, however experienced they think they may be, who is considering teaching disabled people to water ski, is strongly advised to study this first.

The Association now has a nucleus of coaches with experience of training the disabled to water ski, and hopes to build up a stock of some of the devices and aids so far developed. Improperly constructed or wrongly used, these aids can become more of a hazard than a help. Before their use is attempted it is absolutely essential to get in touch with the Association. A golden rule is that when any such devices are used, however fail-safe they may appear to be, or when a blind person is skiing, a quick release should be incorporated in the tow-line which can be operated by the observer in any emergency.

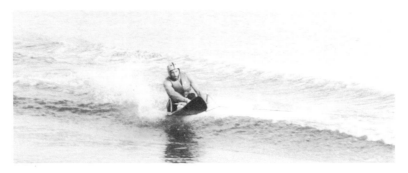

The Sitz Ski enables Frank Jespers, a paraplegic, to enjoy the thrills of water skiing.

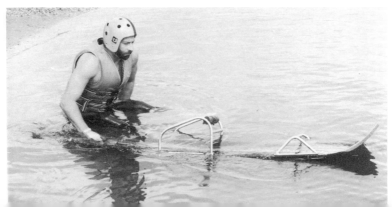

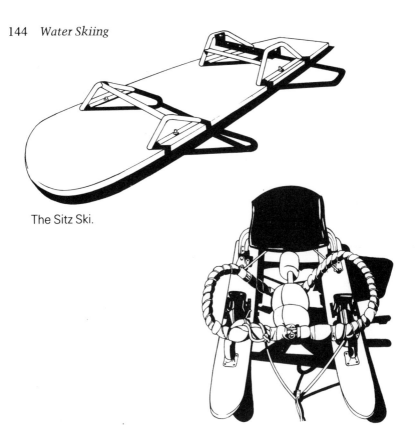

The Sitz Ski.

The American Ski-Seat with shaped seat and protective cushioning.

THE FUTURE

At present there is rapid advancement in the achievement of disabled water skiers. There seems to be no form of the sport which cannot be mastered by the determined disabled water skier with only three usable limbs, or possibly even greater handicaps. Jumping, slalom, trick or figure skiing, barefoot skiing and para-kiting have all been achieved by disabled water skiers. Such accomplishments show that the sport need not be limited to simply following a boat round a lake. It can encompass a broad and exciting range of activities.

Close contacts are being established with the Disabled Water Skiing Section of Group II in Europe (to which the British Water Ski Federation belongs) and no doubt there will eventually be competitive events both on a national and international scale.

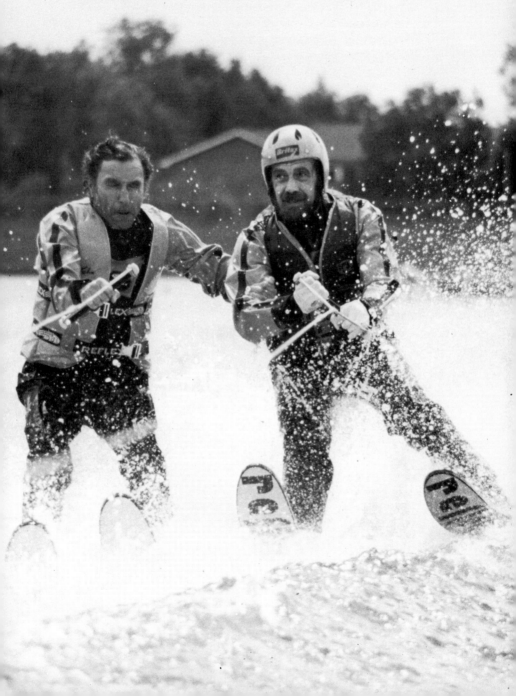

Nigel Verbeek (right) being guided over the wake of the boat by instructor Peter Felix.

Nigel Verbeek is a blind water skier who came to the sport by chance:

'Blind faith — yes, that's the basis of water skiing when you are blind. Faith in your driver, your instructor and equipment. A chance meeting at a party with a very competent water skier led to an invitation a few months later to join him at Princes Water Ski Club. In a moment of madness I agreed. Duly kitted out in borrowed wet suit, lifejacket and skis, a first conventional attempt was, needless to say, disastrous — arms, legs and skis everywhere plus a bellyful of not too appetising water. The second attempt fared little better, but the third, with the aid of a long pole, in place of a conventional handle, borrowed from the B.D.W.S.A., allowed me to be sandwiched between two expert skiers who with no trouble, on the very first attempt, lifted me onto my skis and enabled me to sample that tremendous exhilaration. I was well and truly hooked.

Progress from here was rapid. I had soon dropped one of the instructors and, in tandem only, proceeded to mono-ski, cross wakes, deep water start, jetty start on one and two skis and eventually progress to the single handle while my instructor skied alongside on a separate line for directional purposes.

Barefooting was the next challenge and success was not long in coming, albeit for only a few seconds, on a barefoot bar attached to the side of a boat at the B.D.W.S.A. meeting at Holme Pierrepont. Following this, several attempts were made at the deep water start but as yet my best is ten seconds standing.

Next came jumping, again on two separate lines, with an instructor to direct me to the jump and valuable advice from Paul Seaton and Peter Felix. Although the run and jump were satisfactory, the landing was a shambles, but I am still working on it. During the coming season I promise myself not only the satisfaction of landing after jumping but also that barefoot badge for half a minute on my feet.

Yes, it is a tremendously exhilarating sport to be enjoyed by the blind as well as many other disabled people alongside their non-handicapped colleagues.

Yes, I am really grateful to Irving Stone for that chance meeting at a party which led to my introduction to this great sport.'

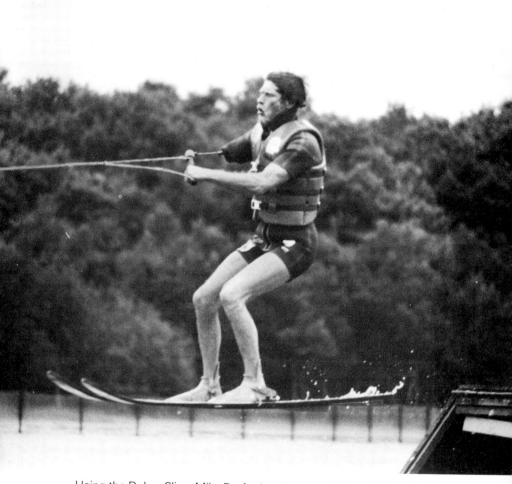

Using the Delgar Sling, Mike Bayford makes a good take-off from the ski jump.

Mike Bayford, a one-armed water skier, describes how a simple aid opened up new possibilities in the sport:

'Although it is quite possible to water ski unaided using only one arm nevertheless it is very tiring, limiting skiing time, and it took two years of sheer desperation to achieve a deep water start on a mono-ski, nearly pulling my good arm out of its socket in the process.

The discovery of the Delgar sling completely revolutionised water skiing for me. At last I was able to deep water start easily on a mono and ski for as long as I liked without tiring. I can now successfully go through the slalom course, make the jump and barefoot ski. The potential is almost limitless and skiing at least up to club competition standard should be quite possible.

Although the Delgar sling is a fail-safe system, it must be properly fitted and designed to work safely and satisfactorily, but as it is attached to the body, it is a golden rule of the B.D.W.S.A., through whom I can be contacted for advice, that a quick release must always be used on the boat.

It is one of the strange twists of life that, although I lost my arm round a propeller while snorkelling, water skiing behind a motor boat is now my favourite water sport. In fact now, in tandem, I can even lift out a one-legged water skiing friend of mine. Three-armed, three-legged water skiing!'

12. Power Boating

Power boating has caught the public eye and the headlines in recent years through the development of offshore power boat racing, first in America and then in Britain. Power boat racing is closely allied to motor racing with its high speed and its demand for special hulls and engines which are pushed to the limit in championship meetings; but it is only one aspect of a sport which has many facets, and which can offer much enjoyment and fulfilment to disabled people.

At one end of the range there is the small dinghy or inflatable, equipped with a 1 or 2hp outboard motor, while at the other end popular power boating is usually river and estuary cruising in heavy craft with powerful marine engines. Between these contrasting power-assisted boating activities are a number of fascinating sports such as water skiing, sub-aqua diving and off-shore fishing which require the help of competent power boat handlers.

The inflatable is particularly suitable for disabled people because of its stability and buoyancy. Transfer to it is often easier than to a rigid-hulled boat and its buoyancy tubes tend to keep passengers in the centre of the craft. There are no hard surfaces or abrasive edges, and its ease of transport makes it an ideal boat for pleasurable excursions. Sizes vary from the small one- or two-man dinghy which can be equipped with oars and rowed, to larger craft with powerful outboard motors and adaptable for fishing, diving and pleasure boating on rivers or inshore waters.

Whether he is handling a small motorised dinghy or a river cruiser, the driver spends a considerable time in one position. Some movement is required of course, especially when casting off or slipping moorings, making fast, or refuelling — or in an emergency — but many handicapped people can easily cope with these restricted movements.

Controls can be adapted in much the same way as in a car for disabled people. Remote controls can often be installed, reducing still further the need for moving about the boat. Simple adaptations to tools may also enable a handicapped person to carry out maintenance tasks or emergency repairs should these be necessary. Disabled car drivers may also be able to help launch and recover power boats by reversing the trailer down the slipway or beach while the crew secures the bow.

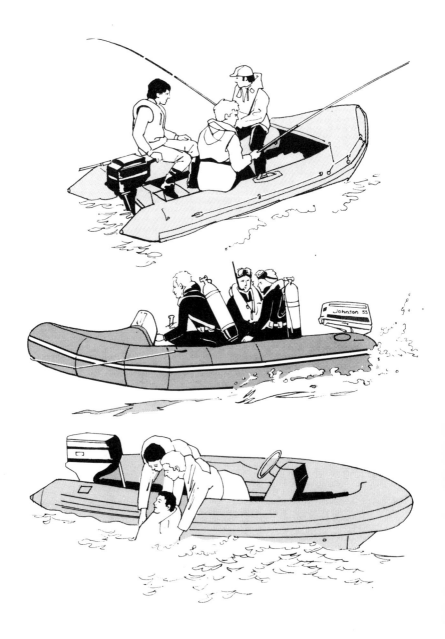

Inflatables are used for fishing, diving and rescue.

The greatest obstacle for would-be power boating enthusiasts is often the enormous cost of boat, engine and trailer. Maintenance costs, servicing and repairs also add to the expense. Sharing schemes, hire and friendly contacts can be explored as ways of obtaining initial experience. The majority of disabled participants probably prefer their water sports to be leisurely and peaceful, free from engine noise and fumes from fuel and exhaust. There are exceptions, however, and if one's personal choice is to join the power-loving, frequently fast-moving and wide-ranging water sports enthusiasts, it is most important to study one's involvement from all angles.

Wanlip Lake, Leicester. Alistair (double leg amputee) and Martin (spina bifida) take the cover off the power boat before launching.

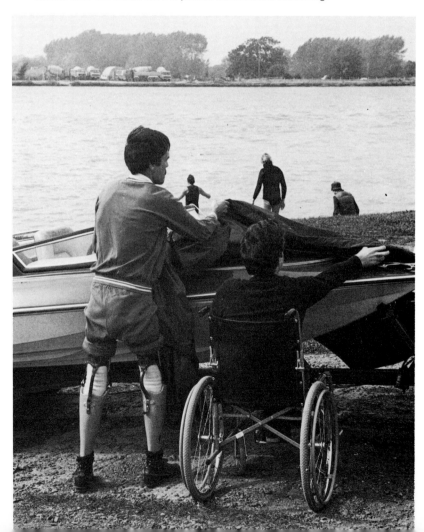

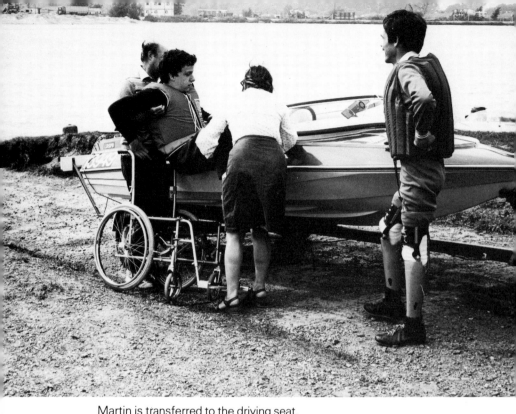

Martin is transferred to the driving seat.

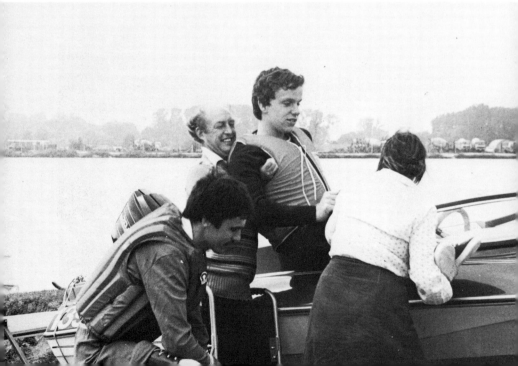

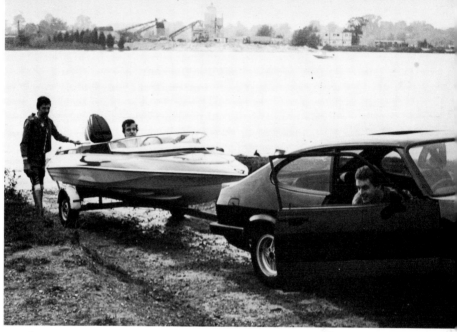

On the trailer on the slipway.

Disabled youngsters enjoying a trip in a powerful rescue boat.

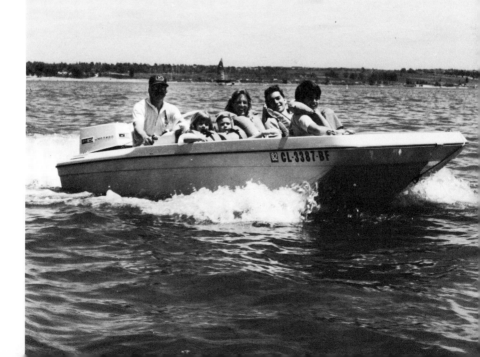

As in all recognised sports, the governing bodies of water sports have drawn up basic rules of safety. Power boat users, and especially handicapped beginners, are strongly recommended to learn the appropriate handling techniques in order to become proficient and competent boat handlers even in adverse weather conditions. This is best accomplished by obtaining tuition at a local club, or a recognised training centre for a particular sport, where the allowances made for disabled trainees are minimal and where everyone has to follow strict safety procedures. Nothing inspires confidence more than obvious practical ability supported by a recognised certificate of competence.

Experienced boat drivers tow water skiers, take teams of sub-aqua divers out to dives, and know how to hold a steady course when controlling a power cruiser in choppy water. There is also a link between power boating and sailing; sailing depends on fast, planing rescue boats on almost all occasions. Handicapped boat drivers can become rescue boat coxswains at sailing clubs. For this purpose it is more important than ever to be able to handle a boat in rough weather conditions, since this is when the greatest number of sailing dinghies need skilled assistance. This is also the time when those who think that power boating is easy discover that it demands skill and expertise.

13. Model Yachting

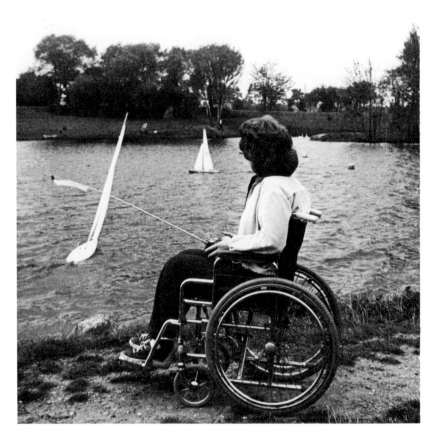

The risks involved in boat-handling are not part of model yachting. Even very severely disabled people are able to enjoy this hobby and compete on an equal basis with everyone else. Radio-controlled model yachts can give immense pleasure. There is a great sensation of involvement as the boat is made to tack, gybe, beat, reach, run and plane, all of which require the same kinds of skill and judgement necessary in full-size sailing. Model yachting can indeed be used to learn these skills for later application in a full-size craft, or it may be regarded as a sport in its own right. The Model Yachting Association has more than seventy affiliated clubs in England and Wales.

RACING

Racing is organised from club level to championships at district, national, international and world levels. In competitive racing tactics are a most important aspect. Normal racing rules are adopted, but because the whole race can be seen in perspective, manoeuvres and tactics acquire a special fascination.

Any stretch of water is suitable for model yachting provided it is at least 600mm (2 feet) deep and free from weed. Races are normally sited round a triangular course of buoys within a 50-metre radius of the operating point. Up to a dozen boats can usually be sailed at one time using the frequencies available, but heats are normally restricted to six.

PHYSICAL REQUIREMENTS

Many disabled people already compete on equal terms with others in this sport. Eyesight and finger control are the most important requirements. There are always able-bodied people available to launch and remove the boat from the water, operations which may be required several times during a day's racing.

EQUIPMENT

Complete second-hand boats are sometimes available through club sources. Kits can be purchased which require little more than assembly. There is a wide range of radio equipment. Two-channel radio is all that is necessary for competition. One channel controls the sail winch and the other operates the rudder. Single-channel equipment with steering only can, however, give a pleasurable sail with any form of model, and many small models are sailed in this way. There are clubs and magazines to give advice to enthusiasts. Like model aero flying, model yachting appeals to young and old alike, and especially to those with active minds and some practical ability.

The Model Yachting Association (see Appendix 4, p.250) will provide further information about the sport and advise anyone who is contemplating taking it up.

A similar organisation, the Model Power Boat Association, also exists to encourage and control activities involving model power boats.

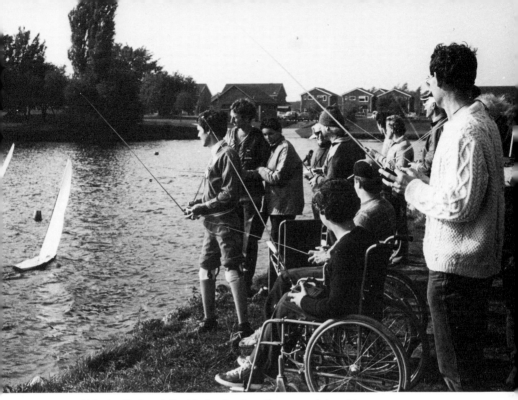

Able-bodied and disabled enjoy together a model yacht race.

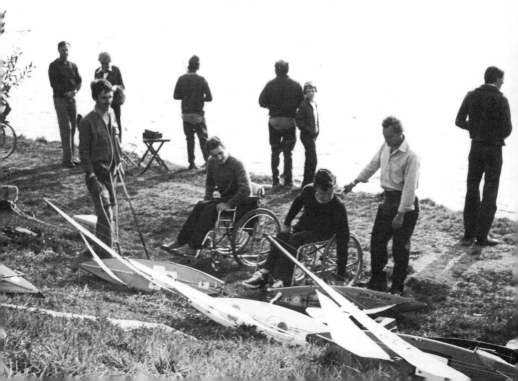

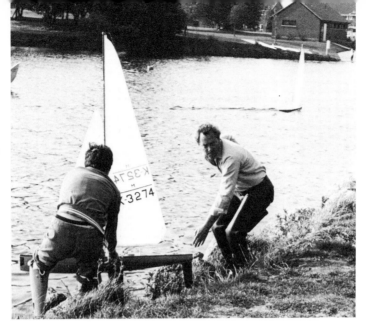

Launching. The youngster on the left does not mind getting his artificial legs wet.

Left: Chris, a tetraplegic, ready to launch his yacht.
Right: Last touches before the race.

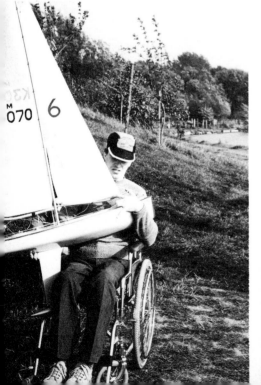

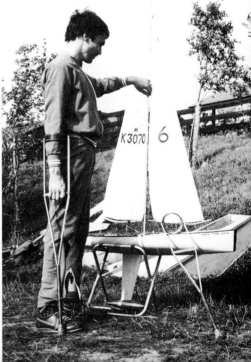

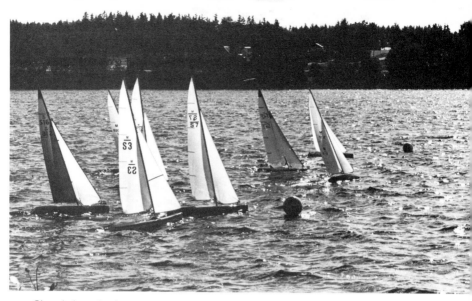

Closely bunched as they come up to the mark.

Typical modern design model yacht with radio-control equipment.

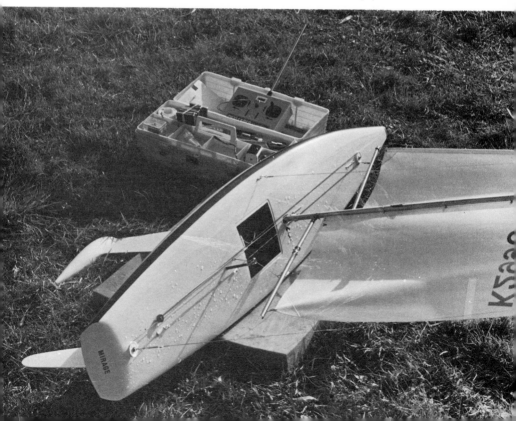

In October 1980 Lynn Moers was cleaning up after a storm. A tree fell on his neck and in that one second Lynn became paralysed from the neck down, requiring a mechanical device to help him breathe. He is mobile only with his electric wheelchair, which he operates with a mouth-activated control.

Married, with two sons, he was determined to find an activity he could share with them. The Regional Spinal Injury Center of Craig Hospital, Colorado, U.S.A., explored every option. Model cars proved difficult and cumbersome to manage. Model airplanes were eliminated because of Lynn's limited range of vision and inability to turn his head from left to right. Radio-controlled yachting appeared a viable option if the controls could be modified.

Lynn Moers operates his radio control by mouth.

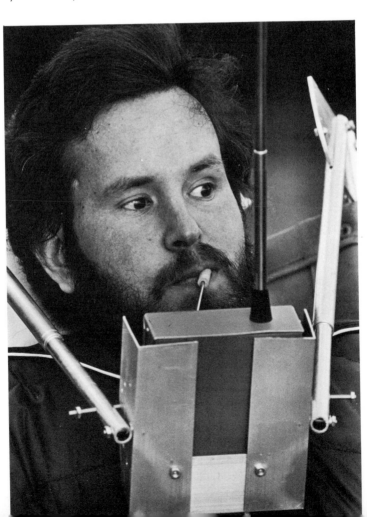

With the help of an enthusiastic expert in model yachting and a co-operative manufacturer a suitable boat was found along with a control which Lynn could operate with his mouth to adjust both the rudder and the sails. There was one further problem — Lynn could only operate the controls if someone stood behind him and held the control box. It was solved by the construction of a tripod type assembly. This assembly, attached to the wheelchair, would hold the control box near Lynn's chest and allow him to operate the controls without help.

'It's a joy,' said Lynn. 'It gives me independence — I was very active before my injuries, participating in basketball, bowling and golf. Now I can get back into a sports activity on a competitive level.'

The attachment to his wheelchair allows him to participate independently in model yacht racing.

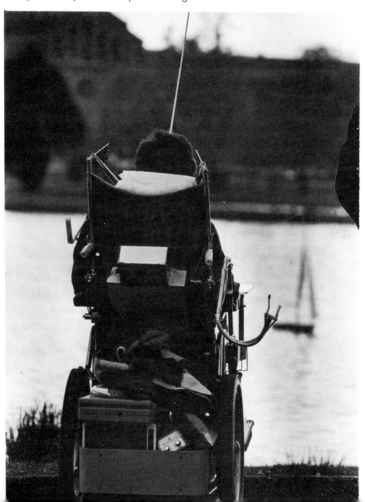

14. Other Boating Activities

Quite separately from the main water sports, many disabled people, like their able-bodied friends, derive enormous pleasure from just being on the water. There is a whole range of informal water activities. Some are strenuous, while the main attraction of others is that they offer the chance to laze about. Boating in the local park, for example, is enjoyed by many people of all ages.

Inflatable rubber boats, such as those used for rescue duties, are particularly suitable for some disabled people. They provide a minimal chance of abrasion and bruising. They are comfortable and offer the excitement of speed. Here again there is a need for a thoroughly competent driver and safety precautions. Lifejackets must be worn. Rubber craft, including air beds, can be extremely dangerous, particularly on moving water, and disabled people must be particularly alert not to put themselves or other people at risk by using them carelessly.

Coracles have been handled very successfully by some people with only one arm.

CANAL CRUISING

For those disabled people unable to handle small boats and water sports equipment, canal cruising provides a delightful recreation. There are numerous canals and inland waterways, and exploring them in one of the many stable craft to be found on them today is an excellent open-air activity. It is suitable both for the lightly disabled, who can help the crew to work the locks, and for those who are totally immobile and may have to be transferred on board on stretchers so that they can enjoy a few hours of relaxation afloat.

Numerous types of craft ply the waterways, but 'narrow' boats provide facilities which are most suitable for disabled people. These traditional vessels are about 12 metres (40 feet) long and nearly 2.2 metres (7 feet) wide, and are driven by powerful, low-noise engines underneath the stern deck. Most of them are privately owned either by individuals or by syndicates, which means that arrangements must be made with the owners to take disabled people for trips.

At many inland waterways centres and marinas canal boats are available for hire, although bookings are usually for at least a week, and seasonal charges for these well-equipped craft are of hotel proportions. Organisations catering for disabled holidaymakers can, however, take advantage of group bookings and arrange either a series of day trips or a journey which involves spending several nights on board.

There are now a number of organisations which have adapted canal cruising boats especially for handicapped users. For example the Peter Le Marchant Trust (see Appendix 4, p.250) was established to give free trips on inland waterways to groups of handicapped people and the seriously ill. People of all ages, including the most severely mentally or physically disabled, are catered for. Demand has proved so great that there are now three boats.

Two are 70-foot narrow boats. One is fitted out as a holiday boat and includes shower, large toilet area, central heating, individually contained cubicles, reading lights, lockers and shelving. Tables, chairs, beds and space for wheelchairs have been designed into the boat. There is a fully fitted modern galley including refrigerator, full-sized cooker etc. For ease of access, there is a hydraulic lift between deck and cabin capable of taking stretchers, and there are also ramps for easy boarding.

The other narrow boat is an open-plan craft equipped for day cruising. It also has a hydraulic lift and a large walk-in or wheel-in toilet and shower area. Good seating, large low windows and good galley facilities make this an ideal boat for a day's cruise on some of the finest waterways in the East Midlands of England. Running hot and cold water and full central heating add to the comfort. A third (broad) boat of 65 feet came into use in 1981. All the boats are equipped with radio telephone in case of emergency.

Another example of canal cruising facilities provided for disabled people is in mid-Wales, where a section of the Montgomery Canal has been cleared by the Montgomery Waterway Restoration Group. This makes possible a total trip of up to six hours which passes through four locks. The *Heulwen-Sunshine* is a warm covered boat with heating installed. It can accommodate eleven handicapped people accompanied by up to nine helpers. Staff and patients can sit comfortably at individual tables and chairs and view the canal through large clear windows. There is also an open area at the bow where visitors can stand safely outside if they so wish. Along the banks the vegetation is abundant and splendid in colour from spring to autumn. Water voles, hares and rabbits, and the occasional fox or snake can be seen. Kingfishers and herons have been sighted as well as unusual ducks and geese, including the colourful mandarin, bred at a canalside farm. The water is rich in fish.

The boat was funded by the Prince of Wales Committee and the Variety Club of Great Britain and is supported by voluntary contributions. Its use is

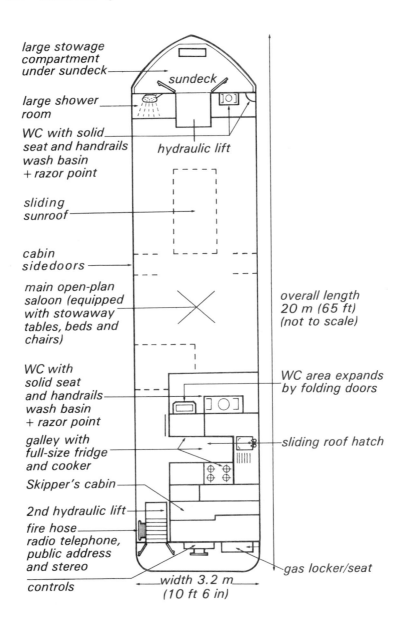

large stowage compartment under sundeck

sundeck

large shower room

WC with solid seat and handrails wash basin + razor point

hydraulic lift

sliding sunroof

cabin sidedoors

main open-plan saloon (equipped with stowaway tables, beds and chairs)

overall length 20 m (65 ft) (not to scale)

WC with solid seat and handrails wash basin + razor point

WC area expands by folding doors

galley with full-size fridge and cooker

sliding roof hatch

Skipper's cabin

2nd hydraulic lift

fire hose

radio telephone, public address and stereo controls

gas locker/seat

width 3.2 m (10 ft 6 in)

The greater width of the canal boats designed for the Peter Le Marchant Trust allows special facilities for use by disabled people.

therefore free of charge to hospitals, schools and organisations concerned with the handicapped. A full time captain and crewman are on board. (See Appendix 4, p.250, for further details.)

The *Kingfisher*, a 60-foot narrow boat for use by people in wheelchairs has also been designed and built for the Spinal Injuries Association. Operated by Willow Wren Hire Cruisers (see Appendix 4, p.250) the boat is available for holidays on canals and rivers in the English Midlands. It is designed to sleep six people. Its features include two hydraulic lifts which can be operated from a wheelchair, a specially designed ramp for getting from ship to shore, extra-wide doors, and a galley and toilet with easy access. It is probably the first narrow boat in the world built to be skippered from a wheelchair.

A family boat, equipped with special facilities for a disabled family member, has also been designed by Midland Luxury Cruisers (Stone, Staffs). It can be booked in the normal way through the firm of Blakes (see Appendix 4, p.250). The *Doubloon* sleeps four to six people, but has an access ramp to the bow deck and an electric lift from bow deck to cabin level. There is also free access throughout the cabin for wheelchairs. Central heating has been instal-led, and there are special adaptations to the toilet and shower accommodation to make them easily usable by a disabled person.

These highly successful examples of planning and adaptation have en-abled numbers of disabled people to enjoy and appreciate the charm of inland waterways. There are encouraging signs that these steps are being followed by other groups and organisations. It is hoped that a time will come when facilities of this kind will be more widely available. A grant from the Silver Jubilee Trust, for example, has enabled the Leicestershire Council for Volun-tary Youth Services to initiate a scheme in which a specially designed canal boat, the *Sunbeam*, manned by volunteers, operates daily trips from May to October. Similarly the Seagull Trust, patterned on the Peter Le Marchant Trust, has been set up to establish cruising for disabled people on the Forth and Clyde, Caledonian and Union Canals in Scotland.

Cruising along a typical stretch of canal waterway.

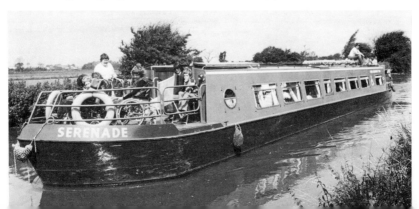

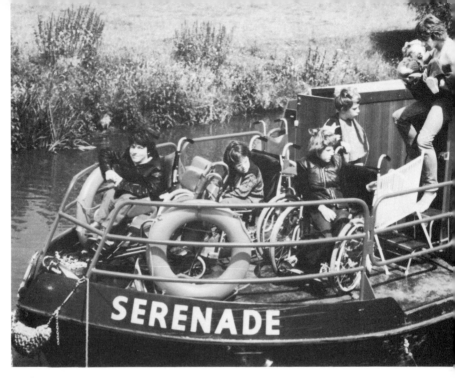

The wide beam gives plenty of room on deck for wheelchairs.

Getting aboard.

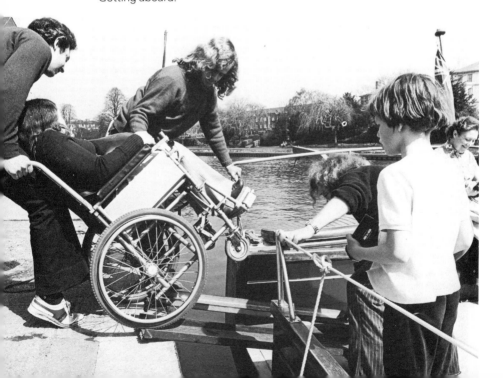

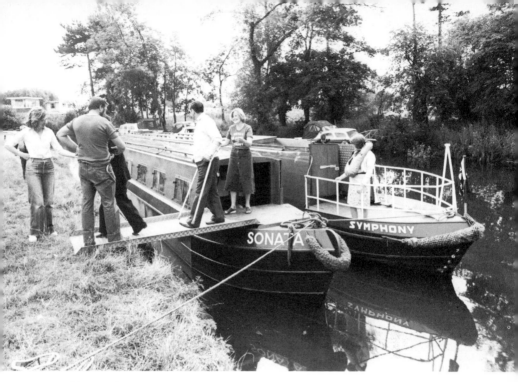

Moored for a break and going ashore.

Going through the locks is always an exciting event.

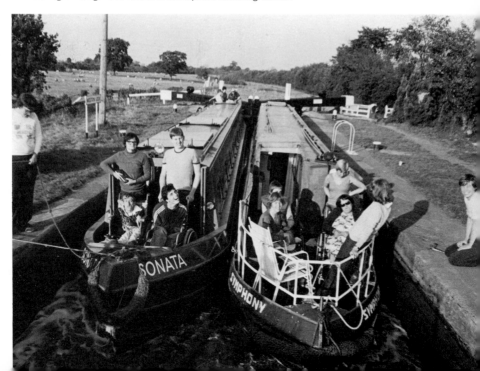

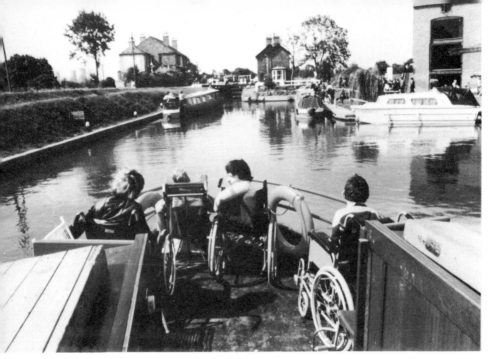

A good view from the foredeck.

The spacious and well-planned galley.

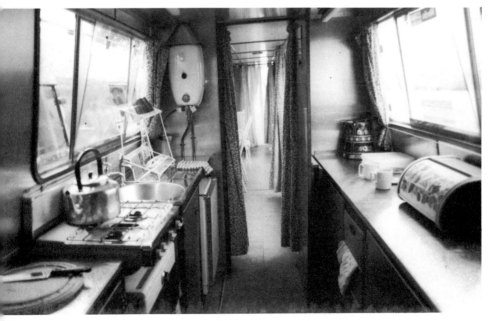

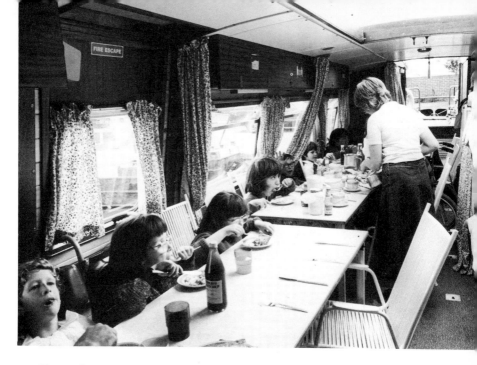

Plenty of room at mealtimes.

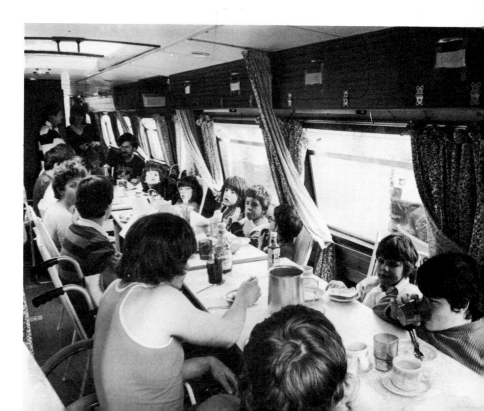

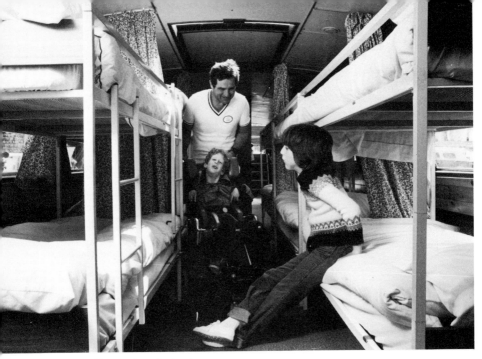

Nearly time for bed.

Willing hands to help get back on board.

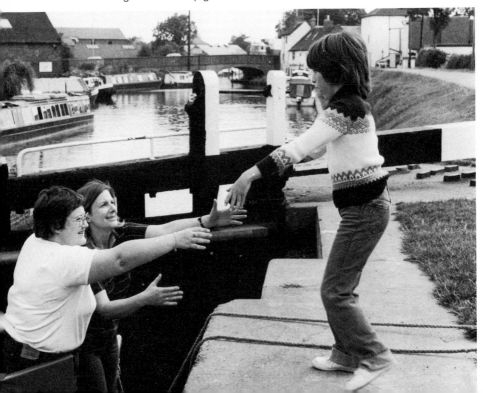

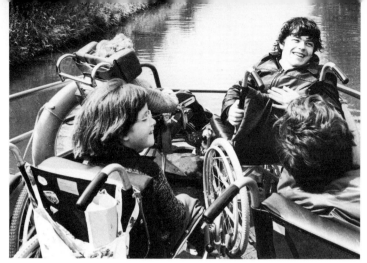

Miles of peaceful waterway.

Sharing a joke.

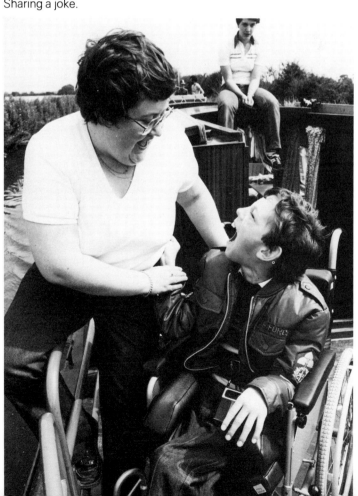

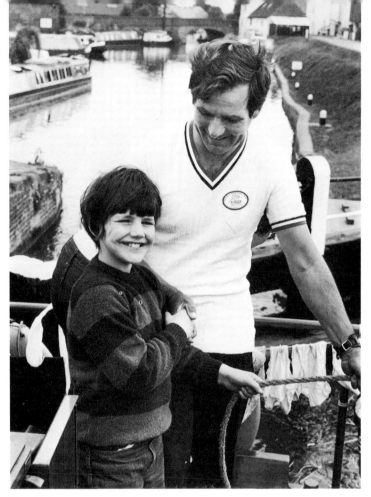

Good friends share a task.

SPARKLE

Sparkle is a catamaran specially built to accommodate disabled people. She is 13.7 metres (45 feet) overall, with a 4.9 metre (16 foot) beam and companionways wide enough to permit up to ten wheelchairs to manoeuvre freely. Participation in sailing activities is encouraged. Commissioned by the First Sea Lord in the summer of 1970, *Sparkle* was built and is maintained by SPARKS, the Sportsmen's Charity. Thousands of disabled children and adults have enjoyed trips on the Thames and from Poole, Chichester and Plymouth. There is a full-time skipper and the boat is freely available to any disabled person. (See Appendix 4, p.250, for details of booking procedures.)

THE R.Y.A. SEAMANSHIP FOUNDATION

The Royal Yachting Association Seamanship Foundation is an educational charity. One of its primary aims is to organise courses or to provide special equipment to enable disabled people to learn to sail and to participate on equal terms with able-bodied people. It has been found that many pupils in schools for the mentally handicapped react in a very favourable way to the concentration and discipline required in sailing a small boat. The Foundation has given a number of small, simple dinghies to selected schools. It also organises an annual course in cruising yachts for up to twenty-four blind or visually handicapped people. Sail changing, anchor work, domestic duties, and all the normal tasks of a crew are taught. A specially developed audio compass enables totally blind students to steer an accurate course. Courses for the profoundly deaf are sponsored, and instruction is provided in other courses.

The Foundation has also developed a single handed trimaran, the *Challenger*, which can be sailed in comfort and safety by paraplegics and other active disabled people who are normally confined to a wheelchair. People disabled by polio, multiple sclerosis and thalidomide, as well as spastics, have successfully tested this craft. The Foundation will provide it free of charge to groups within the United Kingdom, while individual disabled people may also purchase boats for their personal use at cost price. Much interest has been aroused by the possibilities of *Challenger* both in the United Kingdom and abroad.

Specification of the *Challenger*, designed by J.R. Macalpine-Downie.

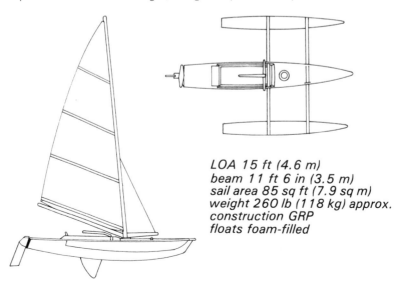

LOA 15 ft (4.6 m)
beam 11 ft 6 in (3.5 m)
sail area 85 sq ft (7.9 sq m)
weight 260 lb (118 kg) approx.
construction GRP
floats foam-filled

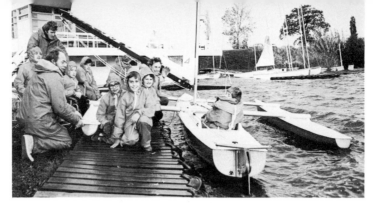

Pupils of the Rose Hill Special School with the *Challenger* trimaran.

The wheelchair can be brought between the floats so that transfer is made easier.

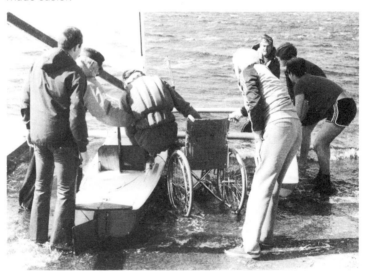

High-speed sailing with stability and ease of handling are the features of the *Challenger*.

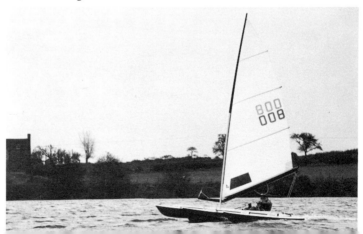

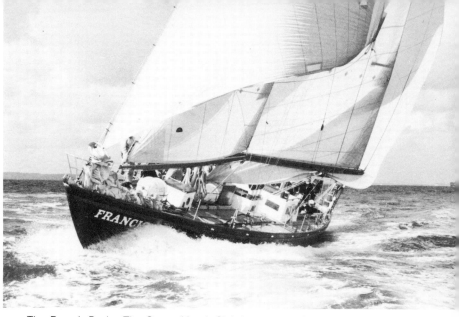

The *Francis Drake*. The Ocean Youth Club has seven of these ketches with two other craft. Disabled people are encouraged to sail as crew members.

Schooner of the Sail Training Association. Crews frequently include disabled members.

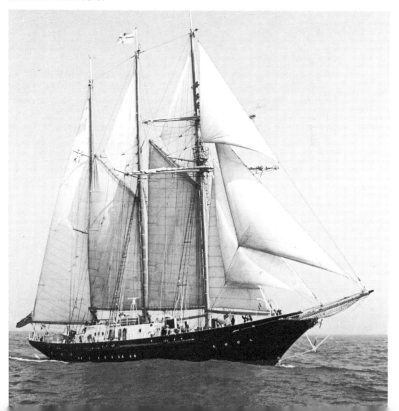

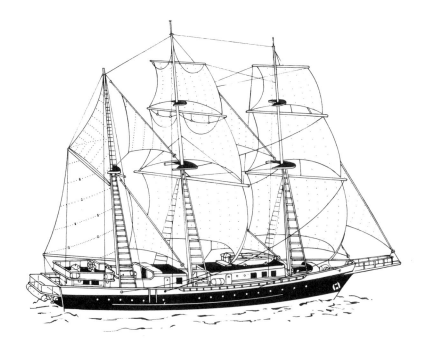

The *Jubilee Barque*. A proposed 135-foot sail training vessel for the
Jubilee Sailing Trust designed by Colin Mudie, in which half of the
crew will be physically handicapped. Features of the design will
include special wide alleyways and doors with flush fittings, and flat
decks with a tracked wheelchair system for the main deck so that up
to eight crew in wheelchairs can be accommodated. The blind will
have an audio compass for steering and the various areas of the ship
will have different surface finishes to help with orientation. A system
of warning lights will be used to alert deaf members of the crew to
orders for handling the vessel. Galley, toilet, sleeping quarters and
other accommodation will be planned for ease of use by the disabled.

15. Swimming

A COMMON DENOMINATOR

Swimming is one of the most popular physical recreations for disabled people. It is often used as a therapy for disablement or for those recovering from accidents in which limbs have been damaged. The warm environment of the swimming pool and the supportive effect of the water enable mobility and freedom of movement which are often difficult in normal circumstances. The emotional and psychological benefits are frequently as valuable as the physical improvements, if not more so.

It is not intended here to describe the various methods which have been evolved for teaching disabled people to swim, or to enumerate the many successful aids which have been devised. Much valuable work has been done by organisations such as the Amateur Swimming Association, the Swimming Teachers' Association, the Association of Swimming Therapy and the National Association of Swimming Clubs for the Handicapped. They run courses for teachers and instructors and have established numerous groups and classes. They come together to pool their ideas in the Sports Council National Co-ordinating Committee for Swimming for the Disabled.

Many useful publications are listed in Appendix 4, and any of the bodies mentioned above will give advice on setting up clubs, the provision of qualified teachers, and teaching methods, as well as guidance on medical considerations and care in lifting and supporting disabled people both in and out of the water.

While swimming is a pleasurable sport in its own right, and there are now opportunities for disabled swimmers to take part in competitions at various levels, it has the added importance of being the common denominator in many other water sports. Many sections of this book have stressed that the ability to swim is necessary before participation in a particular sport is possible. As with the able-bodied, the ability to swim 50 metres is generally recommended

However, it is confidence in the water which is vital. Swimming in the safe, controlled environment of a heated pool is very different from being in cold water out of doors. The capacity to look after oneself without panic after a capsize is more important in sailing and canoeing than the ability to swim a long distance. The disabled person and his instructor must ensure that he has the right lifejacket or buoyancy aid, and the confidence to cope in the circumstances in which he is likely to find himself.

A class for the disabled. Each disabled person has a helper.

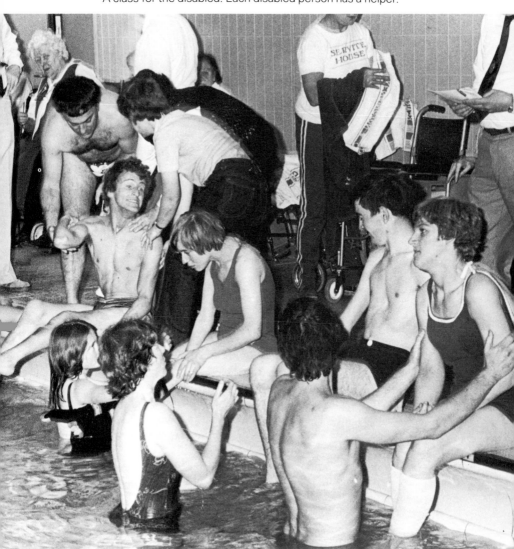

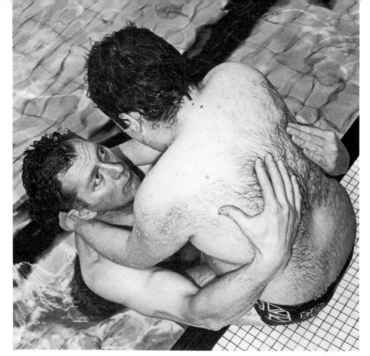

Entry to the water is a major first step. In the early stages quite a lot of support may be needed.

A little more confident now.

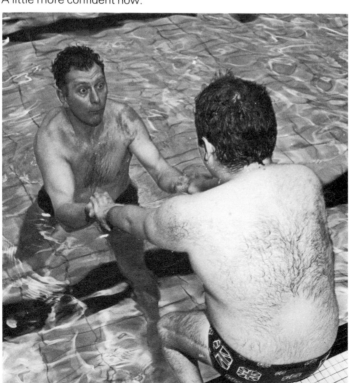

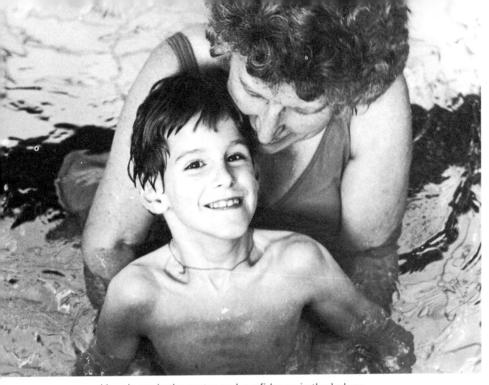

Happiness in the water and confidence in the helper.

Water games to build up confidence, with alternate helper and disabled swimmer.

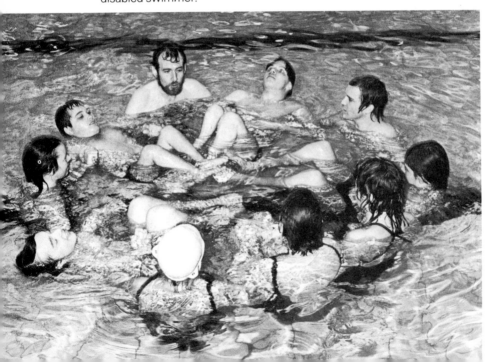

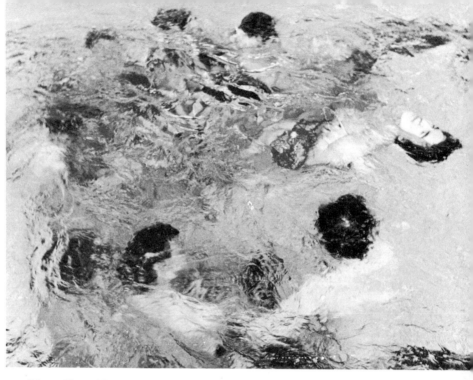

Ring a Ring o' Roses: they all fall down.

The legs thrash through the water like motor boats.

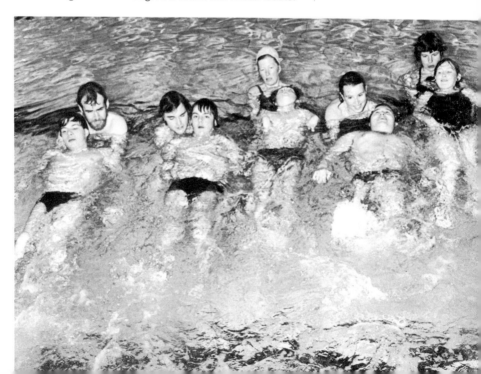

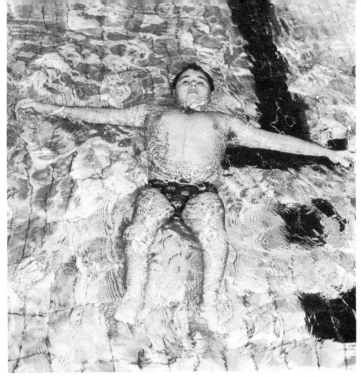

Confidence and relaxation as this young disabled swimmer floats on his back.

Help in getting out of the pool. The hands are carefully positioned to support the weight.

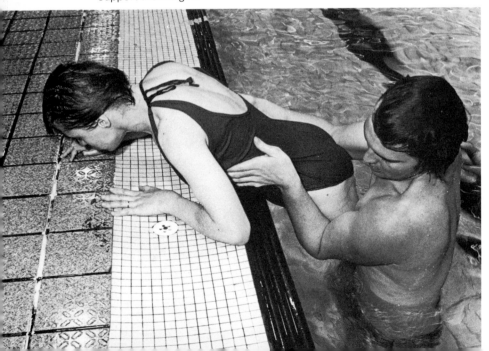

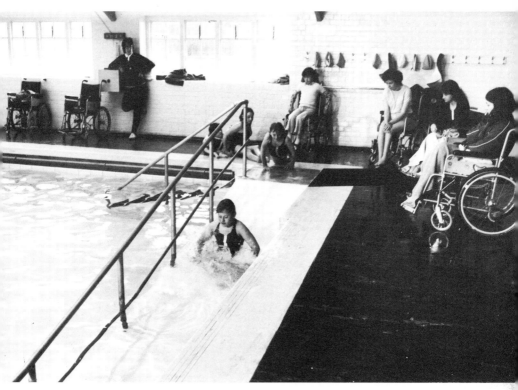

The access ramp at the Treloar School enables paraplegic children to enter the pool easily.

16. Water Sports for People with Mental Handicap

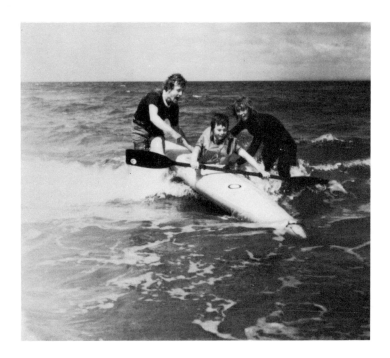

Since the first edition of this handbook, which made little reference to participation in water sports by the mentally handicapped, members of the Water Sports Division have become aware of the unsuspected extent to which activities of this kind have been taking place. The particular problems associated with teaching the mentally handicapped are not underestimated. In general the role of the expert in water sports should be to pass on his expertise to those with special knowledge and training in this field. They can then, in turn, interpret the skills in the terms which the mental handicap and possibly the associated behavioural complications of their pupil demand. Even those with a less severe mental handicap should always have someone in attendance who knows them well.

Swimming, of course, has long been an integral part of the programme for many schools and centres concerned with the mentally handicapped. The Amateur Swimming Association, the Swimming Teachers' Association, the Association of Swimming Therapy and the National Association of Swimming Clubs for the Handicapped have all devised appropriate teaching methods and new courses, as well as stimulating the formation of clubs. The success of their work is very evident.

With this foundation of confidence in the water, enthusiasts in special schools and training centres have not been deterred by the apparent difficulties involved in taking their pupils and trainees out on the water. Their hope has been to kindle an interest and give enjoyment in a side of life which had until then been denied their charges. Often the water sports have been part of a wider range of outdoor pursuits which have also involved camping, fell walking, rock climbing and riding.

In some cases the water experience has been limited to canal cruising using converted narrow boats. *Heulwen-Sunshine* and *Doubloon*, described on pp.163 and 165, have been very popular with groups of mentally handicapped children and adults. The value of this kind of experience, and the opportunities for practical responsibility, are very considerable. Living together as a group; sharing in the navigation of the craft, the working of locks and the sense of exploration of new territory; taking part in an adventure, however simple; from time to time coping with the need to bear discomfort; in the view of many leaders, these activities have often revealed qualities and facets of character of which they were unaware. They have seen their charges in a new light. And if the claims of therapeutic effects cannot always be sustained, no one can deny that the enjoyment and excitement are enough to make the adventure worthwhile.

Motor boating has also proved a popular activity, and the role of the mentally handicapped person can be varied. He may be a passenger, enjoying being on the water, the sense of speed, the wake of the boat and the wind in his face. Or he may, under close supervision, take the helm, handling the wheel and the engine controls, choosing and changing course, manoeuvring alongside and bringing the craft to rest at the jetty. Someone who is mentally handicapped will never drive a car, but on the water he may savour some of the same sensations in safe conditions.

Sailing dinghies and canoes offer a different challenge, and there are examples of these activities being safely practised by mentally handicapped people. The degree of supervision will, of course, vary according to the degree of mental handicap, and it cannot be stressed too strongly that the normal safety precautions must be combined with a special knowledge of the participants involved. It would be foolish to assert that activities of this kind will be generally appropriate, but there is sufficient experience to lead to the belief that, as for the physically handicapped, there is a tendency to underestimate rather than overestimate capabilities. Boldness and confidence have often been rewarded by a gratifying response.

The following examples of successful ventures are given in the hope that others will be encouraged to look around them and consider how they, too, might make use of the opportunities to hand.

BLANTYRE TRAINING CENTRE, ST AUSTELL, CORNWALL

Blantyre is a centre for mentally handicapped adults which offers a programme of outdoor activities including camping, moor walking, forest trails, the Duke of Edinburgh's Award Scheme, sport, sailing and swimming. Various facilities are made available because of the centre's affiliation to the Youth Service, which also provides the necessary insurance cover. The Deputy Head of the Centre writes:

> 'The first problem we encountered in trying to introduce sailing was one of attitude. Some people felt it was not suitable for the mentally handicapped. However, after a few pilot weekends it became evident that here was a programme which encouraged social integration, team spirit and language development, as well as excitement, learning a skill, overcoming fear, and making decisions. As the pleasure and growing skill of the pilot groups became evident, so more students asked to join in.
>
> At the same time we had a swimming programme at the local pool, so students waiting to sail were introduced to lifejackets, water buoyancy and safety practices.
>
> Things have grown over the years, and we now have a sailing boat, a speedboat, a safety boat, the use of a fishing boat and also the necessary safety equipment. Some students do not wish to sail, but they are more than keen to skipper or man the safety boat. Others enjoy the thrill of mackerel fishing.
>
> During the winter months students are busily engaged in maintenance, washing down, sanding, painting, varnishing, greasing, oiling and glass fibre work. We would now welcome an exchange with other centres in different parts of the country which may have developed a range of outdoor pursuits. We feel our students would benefit very much from this.'

Some further details:

> 'We use a wide-beamed local boat called the Celtic for sailing. It is a
> hard-chined wooden boat with Bermudan rig and can carry up to six
> people. Falmouth Bay gives us some open sailing, and the various creeks
> and rivers offer more sheltered waters. Since the tender is very often the
> first craft the students will go aboard, we made sure it was a good stable
> boat.'

COUNTY OF AVON SOCIAL SERVICES DEPARTMENT

Avon Social Services Department has almost one thousand mentally
handicapped adults in eight Adult Training Centres which cater for their
educational, recreational and occupational needs. It had been a long standing
practice that a week's holiday be taken in a holiday camp at the end of the
season. A suggestion was made, however, that rather than take the trainees all
together, a series of small groups throughout the year might be able to enjoy
holidays more suited to their individual needs. Some students found a large
holiday camp rather overpowering. Living in small groups was likely to be of
more benefit.

The past five years have therefore seen the increasing development of
self-catering holidays using an old converted farmhouse in the Brecon
Beacons National Park. This has been acquired as an Adventure Centre by the
Methodist Association of Youth Clubs. A training course was run for centre
staff who would be accompanying trainees. The programme included cooking, housekeeping and general group management as well as the outdoor
pursuits of hill walking, riding, caving, climbing and water activities.

Experience has shown that the optimum group size is between eight and
twelve trainees with three members of staff. Not far from the centre is a canal
where it has been possible to hire a self-drive water-bus for day trips. An
inflatable rubber dinghy has also been used. Encouraged by these experiences,
trips on narrow boats and holidays on canal- and houseboats have now been
introduced.

The manager of one centre says:

> 'Other adventure activities have shown that mentally handicapped
> adults can acquire the necessary skills and awareness of safety factors. I
> believe that water activities will become of great interest to those
> planning recreational programmes. One centre has built a "Mirror"
> dinghy. Staff are being encouraged to take up training courses in sailing
> and canoeing, which, we feel, can be undertaken quite safely and

enjoyably. Of course we would not go out in difficult conditions. Obviously to take part safely in water activities we have regular swimming sessions, and several centres are fortunate enough to have swimming pools on site so that they can build up confidence and safe practice.'

Another manager says:

'It is apparent that the benefits to the trainees from these activities are very great. They complete their "holiday" with the visible signs of personal achievement, and continue to talk of their experiences long after the event. Many are talking to the staff about things they would like to do next year.'

One of the centres describes its canal boat holiday:

'A group of fourteen Lanercoat trainees, along with three staff and a skipper, pioneered a canal boat holiday on the Shropshire Union Canal. The route took us from Walsall to Chester. Initial apprehensions about the danger were soon forgotten when we saw how steadily and evenly the long boat moved through comparatively shallow water.

Two groups emerged naturally. One took the initiative with locking and the mechanics of travelling. The other stayed inside more doing the cooking and cleaning. We glided through beautiful meadows, through small red-brick Staffordshire towns and the urban landscape of the Birmingham navigation.

Evenings were generally spent in welcoming local canal-side pubs. The culmination of our trip was a walk around the Roman city of Chester and a slap-up meal in a gourmet restaurant, where we were given patient and friendly service by the waitresses. At stopping points in the day we had to empty the chemical loos and fill the 200-gallon tank with water. Washing conditions were quite cramped and we found the women were much more particular and efficient about this.

The holiday was not without its light spots: Stephen pushing the boat out and creating a human bridge between the boat and the bank; Richard eating his fish and chips despite a fall and a bloody nose; Mike puncturing the skipper's bike along the tow-path, and the nice but rather naughty film we saw in Wolverhampton.

Everyone was willing to help with the chores, and cooking was amazingly efficient, a variety of enjoyable meals being served. The venture was a great success. We would heartily recommend it to all with a sense of adventure and a care for considerate selection of trainees.'

A further development has been the setting up of the Avon Handicap Adventure Trust whose object is to buy, furnish and equip an adventure centre in the Brecon Beacons for use by handicapped people.

OUTWARD BOUND COURSES

Following discussions between the Disabled Living Foundation, Hampshire Social Services Department and the Outward Bound Trust, an experimental course for mentally handicapped people was held at the Rhowniar Centre in Wales during October 1980. Ten trainees from two Hampshire Adult Training Centres attended. They included some with Down's syndrome and a deaf mute girl as well as some able trainees. They were accompanied by two members of staff.

Before the course the Social Services Officer, who co-ordinated the project, and the two members of staff visited Outward Bound Wales to meet the Warden and the instructors there. This proved of great importance in planning. They in their turn visited the trainees in their centre to see them at work, to make themselves known and to form some idea of the level of disability involved, as well as the nature of the likely difficulties. The cost of the course was borne by the Outward Bound Trust. Valuable help with transport was given by the local Outward Bound Association.

The week's programme included walking, camping, orienteering, climbing, canoeing, rafting, sailing, a ropes course and drama. Together with the necessary personal tasks required in a residential centre, this provided an intensive course for the trainees. Their full participation would not have been possible without the help of groups of six young female students each day from a normal three-week course which was in session at the same time. Thirty-six girls, mainly Police Cadets, were involved altogether and this was regarded as valuable community service training for them. Many friendships were made, and their help and sympathetic approach proved invaluable. One Outward Bound instructor was responsible for the Hampshire group throughout the week, and he quickly established a warm and close relationship. Additional staff were available for such activities as rock climbing, canoeing and sailing.

Assessment of the courses afterwards by staff of the A.T.C.s and of the Outward Bound Centre was unreservedly favourable, recognising that the trainees had benefited both from the physical activities themselves and from the daily tasks required of them.

Comments are vividly expressive of this:

'After tea the trainees unpacked their cases and made their beds, which was a task in itself, remembering that this is not an everyday occurrence for most of them.'

'After they arose they washed, dressed themselves and had breakfast, which they coped with very well. They would then make their beds and sweep the dormitory. They took part in serving meals, clearing tables and occasionally washing up.'

'The swimming and canoeing gave confidence to those who do not have much contact with water and helped to overcome their fears. Two of them were very unsure at first and very hesitant about getting into water. Within half an hour, and with the aid of a lifejacket, they were soon swimming up and down the pool.'

'We paid a visit mid-week to the course to get the feel of the project. We were delighted to see how well integrated into the main course our group were; their enthusiasm for what they were doing, their pleasure in seeing us to tell us how things were going.'

'— they proved to the other students that, given the right opportunities, they can partake in most things that life has to offer in just the same way as their other more fortunate fellows.'

And comments from the Police Cadet students:

'I learned not to try and help them too much or mollycoddle them, but to let them get on and learn by their own mistakes.'

'An opportunity to do something that is completely new to them. Perhaps they have only been onlookers before, but now they can have a go themselves . . .'

' . . . enthusiasm and ability surprised us all and was a lesson on how to make the most of any opportunity.'

' . . . we have all benefited by learning that mental and physical handicaps make no less a person and that determination and a little help can overcome any difficulty . . .'

And what of the future? It now seems evident that the Outward Bound Trust will include a special course of this kind in its future programme and much will be learned from it on both sides. It will also be confirmed in its policy of incorporating, where possible, handicapped students, individually or in groups, in its normal courses and will seek closer liaison with organisations for the handicapped to make this more effective.

NORTHAMPTON ASSOCIATION OF YOUTH CLUBS: THE RANCH ADVENTURE CENTRE

The Ranch Adventure Centre, situated in 11 acres of hillside in the heart of the Snowdonia National Park, overlooks Tremadoc Bay and Shell Island. Nearly at the mouth of the river Antro is Pensarn Quay which was purchased in 1977 for the development of water activities to add to the programme of outdoor pursuits already undertaken. While available to all youth groups, the new centre specialises in provision for young people who are handicapped mentally, visually and physically.

The main social area and all of the bedroom accommodation is on the ground floor, and the buildings have been adapted for the disabled with ramps, large toilet cubicles etc. The safe and sheltered waters are ideal for the handicapped and novice sailor and canoeist.

The Sailing Officer and his team have now built up a wealth of experience of working with handicapped young people:

'As far as possible,' he says, *'we endeavour to use the same boats and canoes for both able and disabled groups, although we have found that Caranoes, because they are more stable, give the extra confidence which is necessary. Fear and uncertainty must be overcome with mentally handicapped youngsters. Even putting on a lifejacket or special clothing may be a harrowing experience. Right from the start we strive to build up their confidence. Tact, fairly firm discipline and good-natured enthusiasm all play their part.*

Both at the getting in, and the once-inside stage, one has to be ready for the pupil grabbing the first thing to hand. It could be the mast, a rope you do not particularly want them to pull, the jetty wall, a spare arm or a leg. But with the helpers strategically placed and the whole operation stage-managed, no harm will come to the boat, pupils or helpers.

In sailing, our routine is to have the coxswain, plus an additional member of staff, to sail the boat. Once the basics have been dealt with, all members of the crew have a go at things within their grasp. Often it is found that someone who has until then shown no real interest in much else suddenly responds to pulling on a rope and moving the tiller. Anxiety and fear can often be dispelled by drawing attention to things happening outside the boat — people on the bank, ducks floating by, etc.

One year after her first trip in a Centre sailing boat June had a trip in a motor boat. All the rest of the group were delighted but not June. She had dissolved into tears. "It's not like sailing," she said. Peter showed no interest in any of the Centre activities such as hiking, climbing, pony trekking etc. He was persuaded to go into a sailing boat. As the boat went about he grabbed the right jib sheet, then on the other tack he did the same. Plenty of encouragement, and for the rest of the week his attitude was quite different.

Even if there is difficulty in getting people out of wheelchairs, we have a boat specially geared up to take wheelchair, occupant and all on trips down the river and out into the quiet waters of Pensarn Harbour.'

Canoeing at The Ranch Adventure Centre. Getting aboard: a wide and stable canoe securely held.

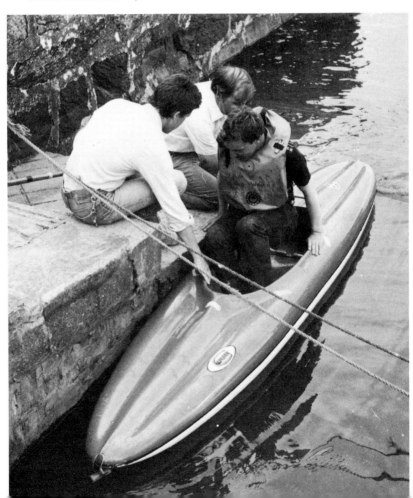

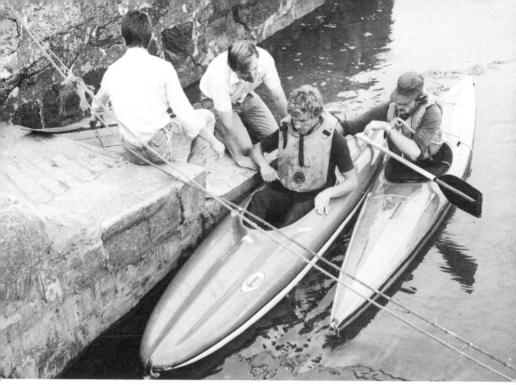

Instructor alongside in canoe gives added confidence.

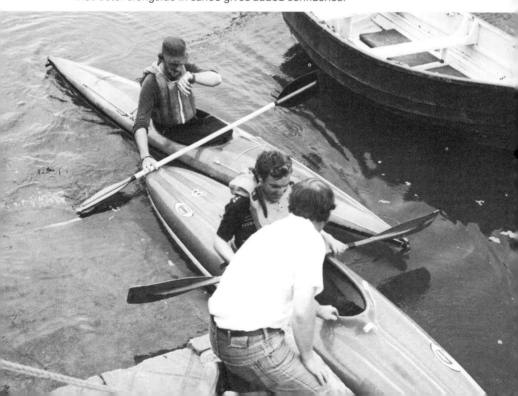

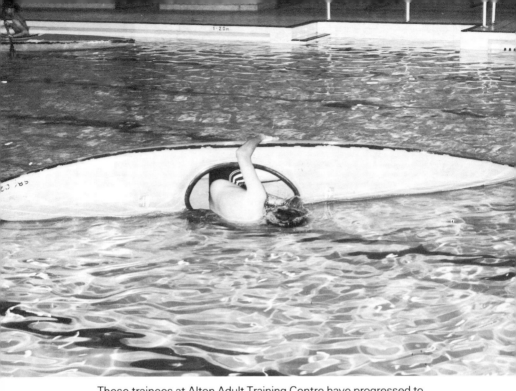

These trainees at Alton Adult Training Centre have progressed to using the kayak and practising capsize drills in the swimming pool.

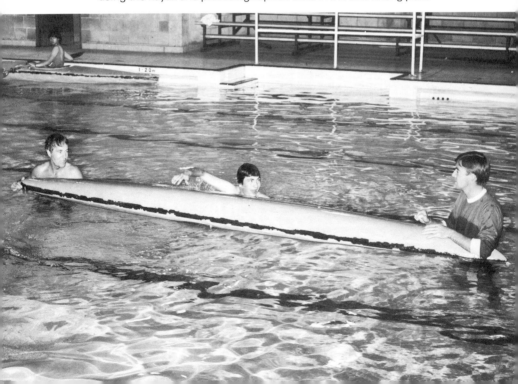

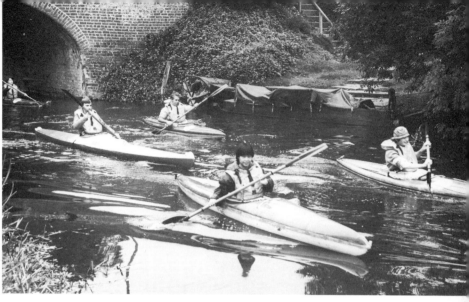

Alton trainees make a canoe expedition on the Basingstoke canal.

Warmly clad and the lifejacket checked before a sailing session at The Ranch.

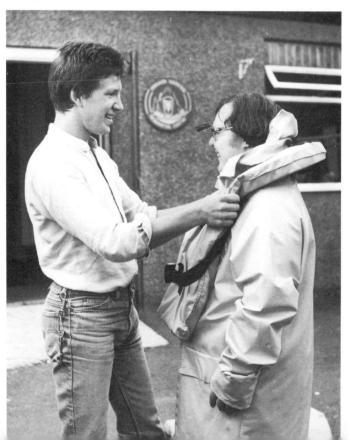

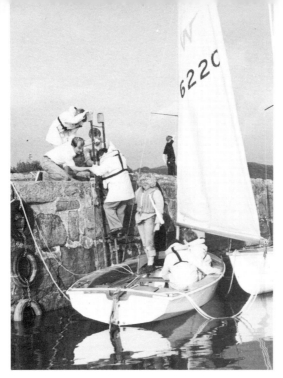

A light breeze only and low water, but getting aboard the Wayfarer from the quay needs some care.

Sheltered water in the bay gives a good safe sail.

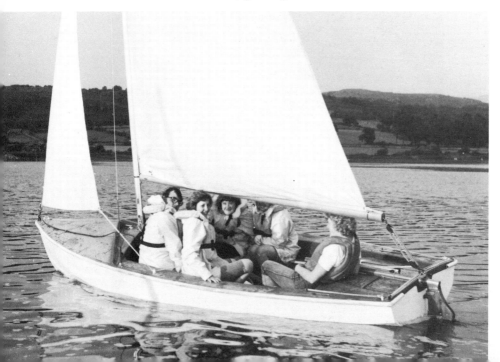

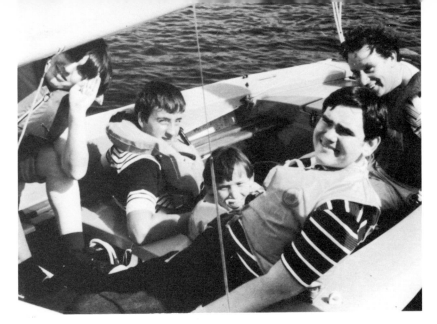

A happy crew.

On a broad reach.

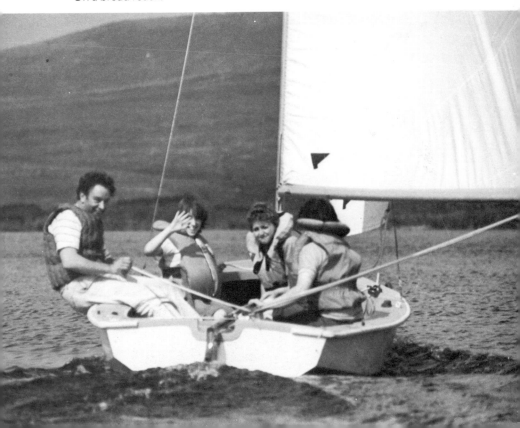

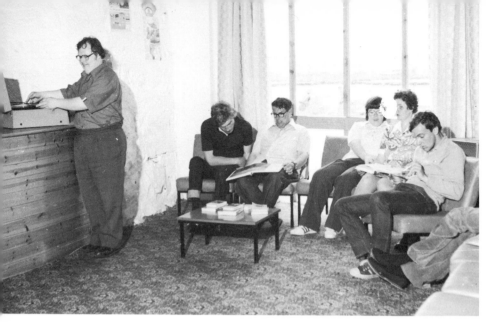

Trainees at The Ranch enjoy a little music in the Common Room . . .

. . . and a chat in the dormitory.

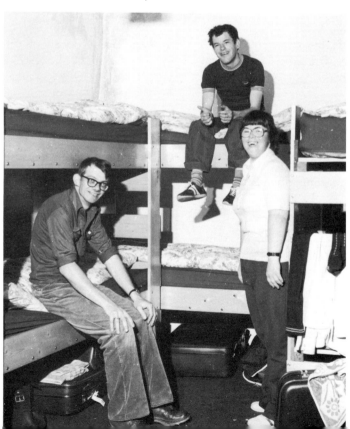

CANOEING FOR THE MENTALLY HANDICAPPED

Canoeing has proved a particularly successful activity with the mentally handicapped. The following guidelines have been produced by the British Canoe Union and will be useful to those who are considering introducing this sport:

The term 'mentally handicapped' covers a wide range of ability. Those at the top of the range can learn in the same way as ordinary students and will just take longer. The less able will need special techniques which are quite simple to adopt and are described here:

Don't depend on words

Some students may not know 'right' from 'left', and instructors using these terms will merely confuse them. The term 'paddle forwards' may be meaningless or may be associated with paddling at the sea-side. In this case it is better to demonstrate, and say 'Do this' or 'Do it like me.' With exceptionally slow learners, the instructor can physically place the blades in the right position and guide the student through the motion.

Free play

Failure to teach forward paddling at this stage should not discourage the instructor. A period of free play, leaving the handicapped students alone to enjoy the activity, will often result in their discovering the technique themselves.

Suitable equipment

Stable canoes, unfeathered blades and skegs make early success more likely.

Suitable environment

Elementary canoeing in a protected area will be sufficiently demanding to sustain the interest of mentally handicapped students for a long time. It is not always desirable to seek more demanding canoeing, as the degree of adult intervention in order to be safe will be much higher. Better to provide a simple activity with a lot of independence.

Timid students

Some will be excessively timid, and will need individual care and encouragement in the early stages. An instructor in the water, holding the bow of the canoe, can keep the boat stable, and encourage the student face to face.

Ambitious students

Some will be unaware of objective dangers, and may not act in a normally expected way. For instance, they may paddle into the path of an oncoming boat and be unable to respond to verbal instructions to come back. This can be overcome by providing sufficient assistants on the water.

Involving specialist staff

Mentally handicapped students will usually be accompanied by staff, or parents, and their co-operation will be invaluable. They may well be taught canoeing alongside their students. Even if they cannot be persuaded to join in, they can give valuable advice at the water's edge about the degree of each student's understanding, and the need for extra care and encouragement.

Small steps

Small steps are the key to success in teaching the mentally handicapped. There is no need for superhuman patience, kindness, skill, or virtue. Ordinary people with ordinary tempers can achieve success if they remember to teach methodically and to be content with small steps.

Individual support and encouragement helps Peter (Down's syndrome) to overcome his timidity.

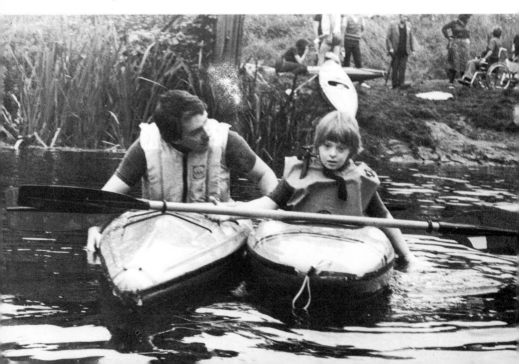

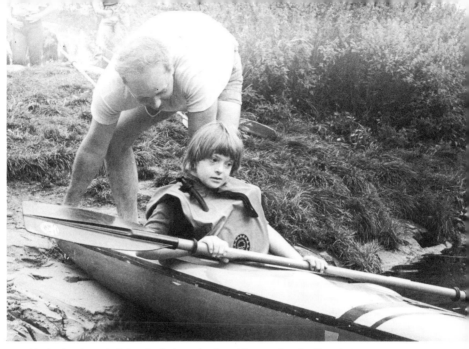

He looks thoughtful as he is launched on his own for the first time.

But there is no doubt about the smile of success!

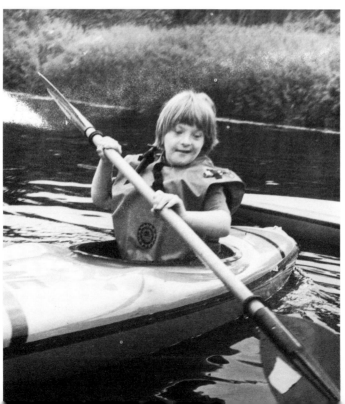

17. Hypothermia

Cold, wet and windy weather can lead to loss of body heat accompanied by a progressive deterioration of body condition known as hypothermia. It can occur quickly and frequently to people who are thrown into cold water and is a danger when participants in sport are in exposed situations without adequate clothing. The condition can develop in its initial stage without the victim being aware of it. Disabled people are frequently at particular risk, since they may not be able to feel the cold in certain limbs. In extreme cases it rapidly results in death unless the symptoms are recognised quickly and immediate preventative action is taken.

The symptoms are:

- Shivering and tiredness.
- A slowing down of pace or effort — though this sometimes alternates with unexpected outbursts of energy.
- Aggressive response to advice.
- Slurring of speech.
- Confusion and abnormality of vision.

Individually, or in any combination, all these are indications of the onset of hypothermia.

People taking part in water sports may build up a 'cold debt'. For example, a racing dinghy crew may capsize two or three times during the course of a race. Each time the body will cool down a little further.

Normally disabled people would not be operating in extreme conditions of this kind, but instructors should be alert to the early signs. Should hypothermia occur, the most effective action is to seek shelter from the wind and to insulate the victim against further heat loss until help can reach him. Additional clothing, even over wet garments, can help. Energy foods and hot drinks could help the victim, and should his breathing stop, mouth-to-mouth resuscitation is vital. Treatment of serious hypothermia is a matter for a doctor or hospital. The essential precaution is that adequate protective clothing should be worn in the first place, and that attention be paid in planning to weather conditions and forecasts.

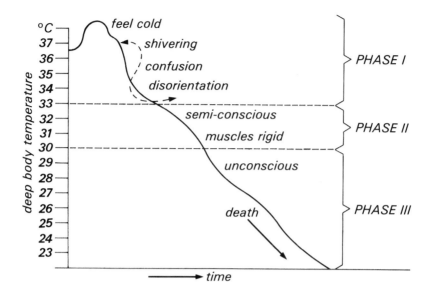

Symptoms of hypothermia. No time scale is given, as many factors are concerned. However, Phase III can occur in as little as 30 minutes in the sea off Britain even in summer.

18. Clothing

Whatever sport is taken up by the disabled, suitable clothing will help to make the activity more enjoyable. Each sport may have special clothing requirements and each disability will require special consideration, but certain factors will apply generally.

THE NEED FOR PROTECTION

Everyone experiences loss of body heat from all parts of the body, though some disabled people are unable to feel that their lower limbs are cold. Others will receive warning signals about this in the form of muscular spasm. This may also upset routine bladder control.

Uncontrolled limbs and insensitive skin areas, usually in the lower half of the body, are liable to cuts, bruises and abrasions. There should be a layer of impact-absorbing, pressure resistant material between the skin and the surfaces likely to cause damage.

Although it is possible to pad some of the corners and frequently used surfaces in special craft, it is usually much more convenient for the user to be protected. Foot and ankle protection is also necessary. It is recommended that the lower half of the body be protectively clothed at all times, even in fine weather. Disabled people who are susceptible to a particular local damage, such as ankle scuffing, should be encouraged to take extra precautions. Instructors should make a practice of checking this at the same time as they check lifejackets.

GARMENT DESIGN

The design of clothing for some disabled people will be affected by the need to provide for incontinence, and to ensure ease of putting on and taking off garments. Women need more fullness in the trouser seat to accommodate absorbent pads and over-pants. Men require a certain fullness in the trouser legs to allow for the wearing of a urine container.

Design for standing and walking is not usually necessary in garments for people with these problems, but wheelchairs make dressing difficult. The fullest use should be made of zip fastenings. People who use calipers should not wear them if there is any possibility of capsizing. However, their protective trousers should allow them to walk about before going afloat and on shore afterwards.

Materials

Two types of material are required. The external one should be water-repellent and resistant to tearing and pulling. The layer next to the skin should be shock-absorbent and capable of conserving heat. The materials should be combined into a dual purpose unit so the wearer does not have to struggle into two garments.

Examples of these materials are 'bukflex' or polyurethane nylon over 'Neoprene' lined with nylon or towelling next to the skin. An alternative inner material is nylon fur, which is very much cheaper than Neoprene. Users should be able to choose either.

The two materials should be fastened together after the garment is made up, possibly with a combination of 'velcro' and zips. The inner and outer can then be separated for washing. Bubble plastic cannot as yet be recommended; it has not proved tough enough to withstand knocks and sudden pressure. The usual bright colours are available.

Design

Although there are several manufactured waterproof clothes on the market, not all are suitable for particular physical disabilities. Looking through the stock of a reputable dealer may produce something suitable. A manufacturer may be prepared to make a special garment to requirements, although this, of course, will tend to be expensive.

Two-piece protective clothing is usually the most convenient. Ordinary battle-dress type jackets with upward-travelling front zips are the easiest to manage. A flat-opening pair of trousers, with zips inside the legs and fork, will be more easily put on and taken off. Heavy duty zips which slide up to the waist from the legs are recommended.

The bootees should be like wet-suit socks, with a zip on the instep. The soles are unlikely to be used. For women, jackets should be styled and where possible trousers should have closer fitting legs. This will give the two-pieces some feminine appeal.

Unfortunately clothing of this type is not yet produced by manufacturers, and it will therefore be necessary to make it at home. Instructions are given in Appendix 2, p.246.

MAKING THE CHOICE

The following more specific points will be of help in making the right choice.

Clothing for water sports should be warm, waterproof and give protection.

Warmth

Even on a warm summer's day it can be very chilly on the water. Fur fabrics are excellent insulators.

Waterproofing

Even if it is not raining, there is a good chance of getting wet from spray. Dry is warm. It is better to be damp with sweat than wet with rain. Waterproofing is thus very necessary.

Protection

Fur fabrics will provide some protection, but if they prove too expensive a pair of under-trousers made from an old blanket will certainly help. Blanket pieces can sometimes be bought cheaply in markets.

With certain disabilities the back may suffer extra knocks. It is a good idea to provide some sort of protection for this area. A glass-fibre 'slope' may be made to fit the back and can if necessary be strapped directly to it. Alternatively a piece of foam plastic can be covered in fabric and tied to the back and buttocks. This gives excellent protection. Additional pieces may be used as leg shields or ankle protectors. A type of closed cell foam sold by suppliers of mountaineering and camping equipment has proved very suitable for this purpose.

Protection of the extremities is very important. The hands must be kept warm and supple. Gloves can be a problem. The feet need special protection against injury and from cold, which can cause great discomfort. Socks made from fur-fabric covered in proofed nylon can be excellent.

Information on many aspects of clothing for disabled people can be provided by The Disabled Living Foundation (see Appendix 4, p.250).

19. Lifejackets and Buoyancy Aids

The wearing of a lifejacket or buoyancy aid, as appropriate, should be a basic safety precaution for all who take part in water sports, able and disabled alike. They serve different purposes, however, and their definitions should be clearly understood. It must be emphasised that buoyancy aids should never be required to act as a proper British Standards Institution lifejacket.

The term *Lifejacket* may only be applied to equipment conforming to all the requirements of the BSI Specification 3595 and bearing the BSI Kitemark. Two types of lifejacket are available: (i) those totally reliant on gas or oral inflation with no inherent buoyancy; (ii) those containing a closed cell foam giving an inherent buoyancy of at least 6 kilograms.

Lifejackets are designed to work fully inflated and will turn an inert body on to its back, in the accepted floating position, in a specified time. Lifejackets must have a lifting becket, an easily adjusted neck strap, and a whistle. They are designed to operate in open water.

Buoyancy Aids are garments, normally a vest or 'tabard', designed to support the wearer in a vertical floating position. They are *aids* to flotation and are not deemed to possess life-saving characteristics. Flotation material varies from kapok to closed-cell foam. Distribution of buoyancy is not defined, so each make has its own characteristics.

Flotation tests carried out with physically handicapped volunteers have been both revealing and inconclusive in their results. They showed that very special care was needed in choosing a suitable flotation jacket which would support the wearer in a working position. Able-bodied persons can combat the designed characteristic of a lifejacket, which is to turn the wearer on to his back. Disabled persons may not be able to.

Legs which have become immobile because of spinal damage tended to sink. Legs affected by polio floated. This may not be a clinical fact, but it was the case with four of the subjects tested. Many of the subjects slipped out of the jackets. This was especially so with a person with only one arm.

Only one jacket remained securely on all subjects. It had been specifically designed for offshore power boating, with a built-in back support and crutch straps. It was uncomfortable and became known as the 'straitjacket'.

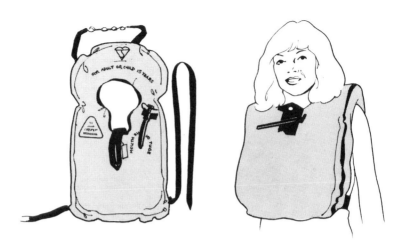

Lifejacket with inherent foam buoyancy and oral inflation to 15.9 kg buoyancy.

Compact lifejacket: inflated orally or by carbon dioxide gas to 15.9 kg buoyancy.

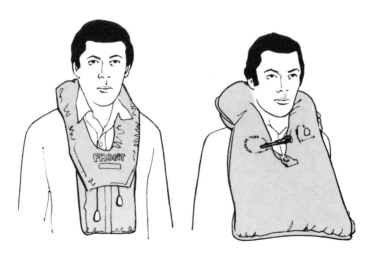

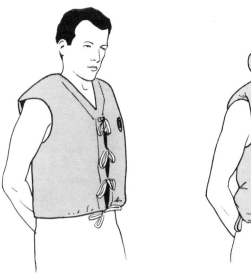
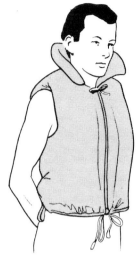

Examples of buoyancy aids.

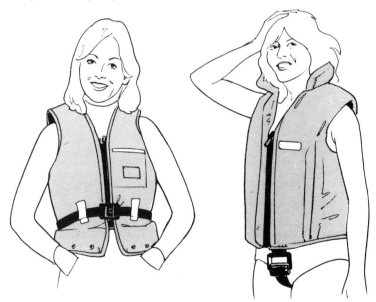

Several points must be considered carefully when choosing a buoyancy aid:

- Can the person support himself in water without a jacket?
- Does the nature of the disability prevent the wearing of (a) a standard jacket, (b) a modified jacket?
- Tests in a pool should be carried out with all candidates to choose a suitable jacket.
- It should be modified by (a) adding crutch straps to prevent it riding up over the head, (b) altering the fastening devices to achieve a snug fit.
- The modified jacket must support the wearer in a vertical position with the mouth at least 100 millimetres (4 inches) above water. (N.B. It is assumed that expert help is at hand.)
- The practicability of combining some form of body support into the jacket should be considered if the wearer has problems sitting in an upright position.

20. Insurance

The importance of proper and adequate insurance cover for all those who take part in sporting activities cannot be stressed too strongly. This applies equally to all participants, whether they be experts or pupils, organisers or helpers. It goes without saying that there are particular hazards in water sports for disabled people. The necessary safety precautions have been emphasised throughout this book. If they are strictly observed the danger of accident or mishap should be quite small, but it would be a very unwise person indeed who omitted to check up on the insurance arrangements.

The following guidelines are set out both for participants themselves and for those who are involved in the organisation of activities.

The decision to participate in a sport must rest entirely with the individual concerned. It is strongly recommended, however, that no disabled person should consider involvement in a water sport without first consulting his own doctor. Medical approval should be a condition of acceptance on all properly organised courses.

Organisers of courses which are specifically for disabled people, or which they are able to attend, must accept full responsibility for arranging adequate insurance coverage.

Insurance should not, however, be regarded as an umbrella covering every conceivable mishap, but as a means of ensuring cover for specifically defined risks, of which there are two types:

1. Being injured or killed (Personal Accident).
2. Being held legally liable for causing injury or death of another person or damage to his property (Third Party Liability).

INDIVIDUALS

Most people have some form of Personal Accident insurance cover. Some, because of the kind of work they do, may also have Third Party Liability cover. Any disabled would-be sports enthusiast not so covered is strongly recommended to seek the advice of a reputable insurance broker and remedy the omission before going any further. It is possible to obtain Amateur Sportsman's Insurance to cover public liability, personal accident, sports equipment and personal effects. Some companies offer this cover to disabled persons, although personal accident cover may be excluded.

It is of course advisable to 'shop around', since the first offer is not necessarily the best.

Anyone who invites a disabled person to take part in a sporting activity, either under his voluntary guidance, or in his craft, should make sure that both have adequate insurance cover to meet the needs of the situation.

ORGANISED COURSES

Local Education Authorities, local authorities, sports associations, governing bodies of sport, voluntary or statutory organisations and clubs, all carry insurance to cover their usual business and activities as well as their officials. Any organisers of courses for disabled people carried out under their aegis must ensure that the insurance cover available extends to include this particular situation.

The Royal Yachting Association, the governing body for sailing in Britain, advise in their *Notes on Insurance*:

> 'There is no substitute for declaring to your insurers everything which you think is likely to happen and to make sure that the individual, the club or organisation have adequate insurance cover for every eventuality for which they might be deemed to have "an insurable interest" and therefore some responsibility.'

Each situation requiring insurance cover is likely to be different. The responsibility must therefore lie with each individual to ascertain that adequate insurance cover is available in whatever capacity he or she is operating. The Third Party Legal Liability section is perhaps the most important in any insurance policy.

Advice on the particular needs of each sport can be given by the governing body concerned. In some cases they may be able to recommend insurance companies or brokers accustomed to dealing with the special situations involved, and who may be approached directly by individuals or clubs.

All regions, county associations and affiliated clubs and schools are included in the Public Liability insurance policy of the British Sports Association for the Disabled. It is essential, of course, that application subscriptions be up to date. The Indemnity Limit is £500,000.

Disabled sportsmen and women may obtain Personal Accident insurance at attractive terms through the British Central Council of Physical Recreation Insurance Bureau. A comprehensive range of death and injury benefits is available. Arrangements can be made for individuals to pay the premium through regional secretaries of the British Sports Association for the Disabled if they so wish.

21. Access and Facilities

WATER RECREATION AREAS

'The freedom and refreshment of being out in the country is just as necessary and enjoyable to the minority of people who are permanently disabled as it is to able-bodied people — perhaps more so. Yet all too often the countryside experienced by disabled people is marred, not by their disability or mobility aids, but by an environment which has been modified by the able-bodied for able-bodied people.' (Informal Countryside Recreation for Disabled People, Countryside Commission.)

River bank footpaths, canal tow-paths, reservoir viewing points, wild fowl sanctuaries, fish hatcheries and pleasure boat bases and pick-up points are some of the water-based countryside amenities which should be accessible to disabled and able-bodied people alike.

Fortunately local authorities, private clubs and other providers of such facilities are beginning to recognise the needs of handicapped people and their potential ability to share in the use of recreation amenities.

Most existing clubhouses do not require a great deal of adaptation to make them accessible for disabled people. Often the best thing is to invite a disabled person to come and give advice on the spot. External doors to buildings are usually wide enough to permit wheelchairs to pass through. Problems are caused by steps leading up to them. When combined with heavily sprung doors, a weather-resisting threshold and a doormat, they will defeat all but the most experienced chair handlers. Gently sloping wooden ramps, either temporary or permanent, with shallow battens or a non-skid surface to prevent slipping in wet weather, can provide the solution.

Doors to changing rooms and toilets are frequently narrow and are further impeded by interior 'modesty' screens. Changing in boat sheds or equipment rooms may be an acceptable alternative, but it is sometimes necessary to provide portable lavatory accommodation of the 'Elsan' type. The main requirements are reasonable privacy and sufficient room for a disabled person and helper to move about fairly easily. The facility may be used by both sexes, and where the spouse is the helper this is essential.

When new recreational complexes are provided, the necessary access

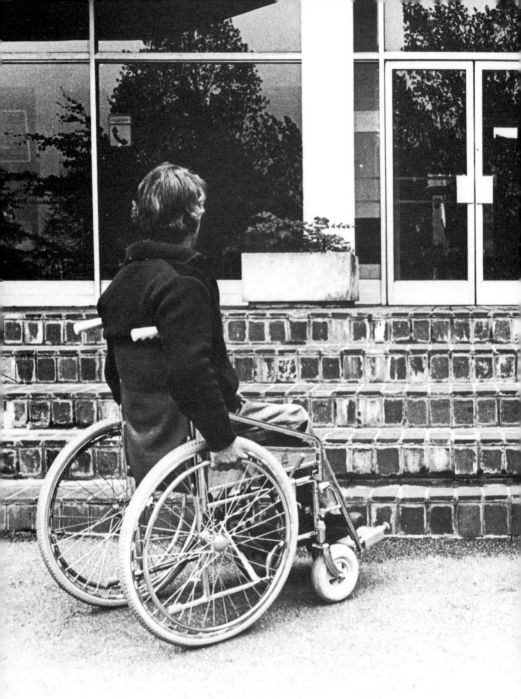

A formidable hurdle to negotiate: five steps to the entrance.

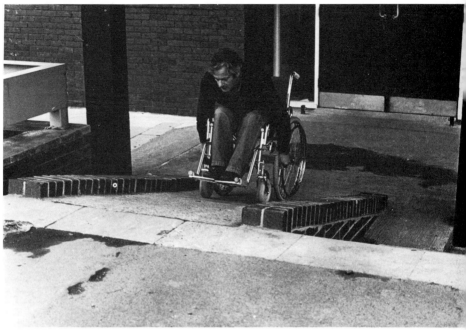

A gradient of 1 in 4 is like an obstacle course in a wheelchair.

Good access with a gently sloping ramp, although the bicycles don't help.

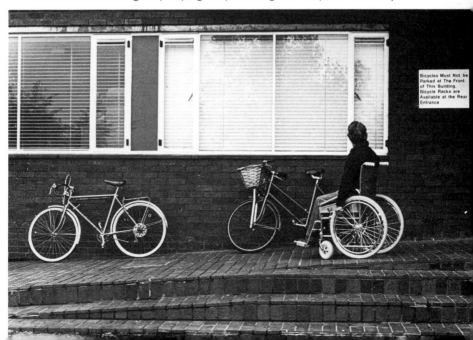

requirements should be included at the planning stage. Consultations between commissioning authorities, architects and representatives of the disabled community will ensure that the facilities will be accessible to both able and disabled users.

ACCESS TO GENERAL FACILITIES

Handicapped sportsmen may be able to walk with or without aids, or they may require partial or continuous use of a wheelchair in all places except when actually in the various water craft. Some of the places where access problems arise are listed below and suggestions made for improvements. It is desirable that there should be easy access between all these areas.

Car parks

Disabled people travel most usually by private transport or in adapted vehicles and less commonly by public transport. They usually wish to be taken as close as possible to the destination, especially when arriving unaccompanied and perhaps with equipment and protective clothing to carry.

The first priority is to set aside one or two car parking spaces adjacent to main buildings, with access points as near as possible to the water. The surface should be hard, level and smooth and of a sufficient width to allow car doors to be fully opened (5 × 3.6 metres; 16½ × 12 feet). A reserved notice or the international handicapped sign is usual.

The dropped kerb to the pavement and gentle ramp with handrail at the entrance give good access for the disabled.

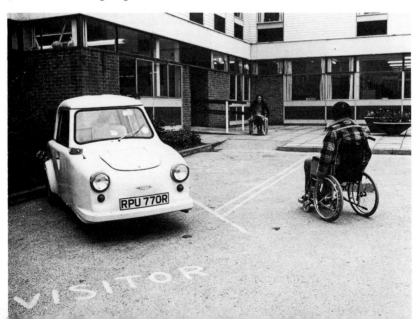

The Stoke Mandeville Sports Centre for the Disabled: broad, gently sloping access and wide doors.

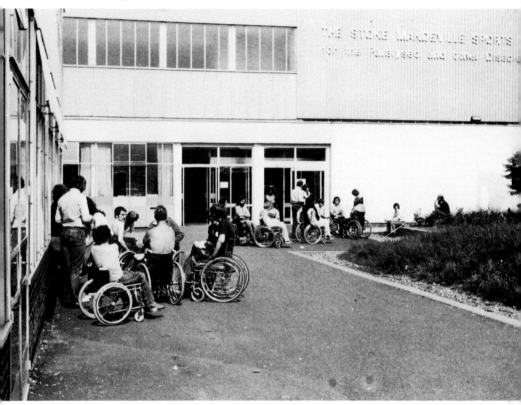

Spectator stands

A number of hinged seats in vantage positions will allow wheelchair users to use the stands without obstructing passageways. They should preferably be under cover. There should be step-free access through entrances and exits, and to toilet and refreshment facilities.

Picnic and play areas

A hard, smooth-surfaced approach, wide enough for a wheelchair (i.e. 0.9 metres or 3 feet) is required. Some level place to sit should be provided and park seats, which should be slightly higher than usual and fitted with arm rests, would be of help to ambulant people.

INDOOR FACILITIES

There are five main areas to be considered:

The entrance

The main requirements consist of a side ramp adjacent to front entrance steps of not more than 1 in 12 gradient, and not less than 1.6 metres (5 feet 3 inches) wide. The steps should have a handrail. Mats should be level with floor surfaces. Revolving doors are particularly difficult for disabled people to negotiate and should be avoided.

Lifts

Public service lifts should if possible be large enough to accommodate two wheelchairs. Lift controls should be within reach of seated persons.

Toilets

Toilet rooms for the disabled may be unisex and should be as recommended in the British Standards Institution Code of Practice (BS 5810: 1979 *Code of Practice for Access of Disabled to Buildings*).

Changing rooms

Many disabled people are naturally sensitive about undressing with others and prefer the privacy of a side room where artificial limbs and orthopedic aids can be left undisturbed.

Because of narrow doors and limited space, most cubicles in communal rooms are inaccessible to wheelchair users. A screened area (3.1 × 2.5 metres; 10 × 8¼ feet) should be provided with coat hooks, mirror, wash basin and shower seat, all at a height convenient for people in wheelchairs.

Social areas

The refreshment area and bar, meeting rooms and offices should be easily accessible for people in wheelchairs.

REQUIREMENTS OF PARTICULAR SPORTS

Getting in and out of canoes, dinghies, rowing boats and other water craft will always present some difficulty for handicapped people, but with help from other water users and by the provision of practical facilities for all to use, the problems can be reduced. Often a little imagination and effort will resolve many of the difficulties.

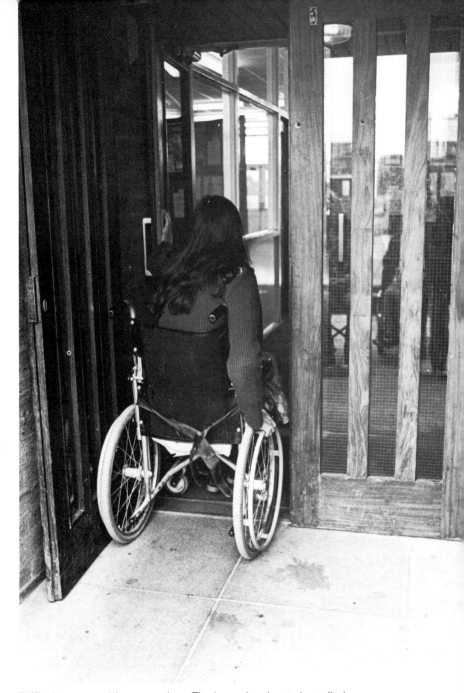

Difficult access with narrow door. The inner door has to be pulled
open and held back. The door mat is also difficult for wheels to negotiate.

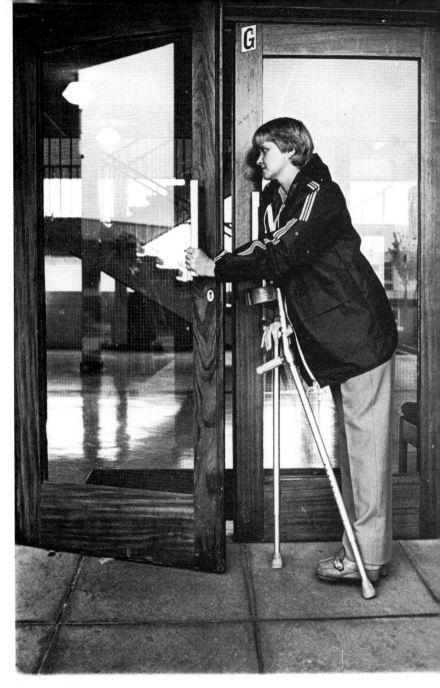

Another difficult access. Opening the heavy door requires a lot of strength and she leans on the other door for support.

Angling

Bankside stations should be flat, and as close to the water level as possible, with a strip of soft ground along the water's edge so that rod rests and sticks can be pushed into the ground. Several small stations separated by grassy areas are preferable to a long continuous strip. Background shelters about 3 metres (10 feet) from the edge are desirable. (For further details see p.27.)

Canoeing, rowing and sailing

Fixed jetties with no steps are better than floating pontoons. They should be not more than 0.45 metres (1½ feet) above the water level; not less than 1.5 metres (5 feet) wide; and they should have a ramped approach. Planks should be across the walkway instead of running from end to end. One of the launching slipways should not exceed a gradient of 1 in 10 and should continue well below water level so that wheelchair users may get alongside their boats and canoes. In tidal water centres most disabled people will use the boat access routes.

Water skiing

Provided there is access to the water facilities from car parks and changing rooms, no special provision is required.

Sub-Aqua

There are particular problems in enabling disabled divers to have access to the water from the beach, jetty or from boats. These are dealt with in detail on pp.113 - 126.

22. Getting Others to Help

There are many organisations and individuals who are in a position to give help in a variety of ways in promoting water sports for disabled people. The advice which follows is intended mainly for associations or clubs which have decided to undertake such a venture. Much will be found here, however, which will be of assistance to any disabled individual who is contemplating taking up a sport.

The governing body of the sport concerned can of course be turned to for guidance and will be able to establish useful local contacts. The Water Sports Division of the British Sports Association for the Disabled is always available for consultation and advice. Through its National Co-ordinator and the regional agencies of the B.S.A.D. it is able to provide information about facilities and courses and to assist in planning.

PROVIDERS OF FACILITIES

The Amenity Officers of Water Authorities are responsible for the recreational use of reservoirs, and will know what opportunities exist there and on the various rivers and other stretches of water which lie within their regions. Some publish pamphlets which give details of clubs, facilities and events.

Outdoor centres sometimes run courses specially for the disabled, or they may welcome a few disabled people on open courses. These centres may be part of the Local Education Authority provision for schools or the youth service but their programme is often open to members of the general public. A number of the national voluntary organisations, such as the Scouts Association, Guides, Y.M.C.A. etc., also possess outdoor centres. Others are independently organised. Over recent years there has been an increasing and welcome willingness to adapt facilities so that they may be used by the disabled, and to include the disabled in the programme of activities.

Sports Council regional staff will be well briefed on facilities available in their area. An approach to them will often prove fruitful.

CONTACTING DISABLED PEOPLE

Disabled people are often unaware of the opportunities which exist in their locality, and making contact with them sometimes proves a problem. Valuable advice on this will be found in the leaflet *How to Contact Disabled People*, published by the Disabled Living Foundation.

The Local Education Authority can help: some Authorities have officers with special responsibility for the education of the disabled. They will know about disabled people in special schools, and also about those in ordinary schools and colleges of further education etc., and in youth clubs. The Social Services Departments have registers of disabled people as well as responsibility for training centres and residential homes. They may be prepared to circularise information about courses and facilities. They are naturally not prepared to disclose details of their 'clients'.

Information about swimming and other sports clubs for the disabled, clubs for blind people and Physically Handicapped/Able-Bodied (P.H.A.B.) local associations, can be obtained from the various national organisations. Lists will often be found in local libraries. Much work with the disabled is also done by voluntary organisations such as the W.R.V.S. and the Red Cross, who will help in making contact.

The British Sports Association for the Disabled, which was founded at Stoke Mandeville, Buckinghamshire, in 1961, is a national association to co-ordinate and develop sport for all disabled people, and works towards the improvement of facilities for them. Through its regional committees and numerous affiliated clubs it encourages participation in all kinds of sporting activities, and gives guidance on facilities, equipment and instruction.

TECHNICAL HELP ON THE MEDICAL SIDE

Physiotherapists and remedial gymnasts recognise the valuable contribution which sport can make in the rehabilitation of the disabled, and towards their welfare. Among them will be found helpful enthusiasts prepared to play a leading role in promoting a sport in which they often have a keen interest themselves. Occupational therapists are also becoming increasingly involved. Approach to them may be made through their national organisations, or locally through hospitals or health authorities.

Doctors may also be prepared to guide their patients towards participation in activities, and to advise on the suitability of certain sports for particular disabilities.

Teachers in special schools and in residential centres can also be counted on to give help. If they participate as members of courses, they are able to play a vital role in assessing the suitability of activities and explaining the medical implications of disabilities.

COACHING AND INSTRUCTION

It is essential to employ instructors who are experienced and highly qualified. Initially they may be experts in the sport but they will require guidance on the special needs of the disabled. This may come from the physiotherapists and staffs of special schools and others with medical knowledge. Instructors can be encouraged to attend the kind of courses organised by the Water Sports Division of the B.S.A.D. This will enable them to adapt their specialist knowledge to the particular disabilities they will meet with. There is a shortage of instructors who have knowledge and experience in both fields, and everything possible should be done towards building up a body of such people.

The regional staff of the Sports Council will provide the address of the local branch of the appropriate governing body of sport. Help should also be sought from the Physical Education Adviser of the Local Education Authority. The latter may have classes for the disabled in its Adult Education Programme. The Adviser will also know of physical education teachers prepared to help, and of the opportunities offered by the various educational institutions in the area. The Recreation and Amenities Officer of the district or county authority should also be conversant with the provision made at sports and outdoor activity centres.

TRANSPORT

The provision of transport for disabled people to and from the site can be one of the most pertinent problems. It can, however, be overcome in nearly every case. Local sportsmen in clubs are often prepared to take disabled friends with them. Voluntary organisations, such as Rotary, Lions Clubs, Round Table and Red Cross will frequently provide this service. Local authority Social Services Departments are also able to transport disabled people for recreation purposes, and there are excellent examples of them co-operating to provide a joint service.

FINANCIAL HELP

The Health and Social Services Department of a Local Authority is responsible for making provision for the chronically sick and disabled under Acts of Parliament. The Local Education Authority also has certain duties to provide adequate facilities for recreation and social and physical training. Funds are inevitably short, however, and the situation has become aggravated over the past few years. There is therefore much call for financial aid from voluntary sources. Lions Clubs, Rotary and Round Table Associations and other similar organisations have proved willing organisers of fund-raising events. These have done much to help get activities for the disabled off the ground, and to support them.

Grants may also be available through the sports development allocation to the Regional Council for Sport and Recreation. Sponsorship by some local firm or organisation has been found, on occasion, to be a successful method of raising the necessary funds.

Helpers are needed for many tasks and the most appropriate and willing are generally fellow sports enthusiasts. Local school leavers, college students, members of the Armed Services, and Police Cadets frequently offer their help in many ways.

EQUIPMENT

In the various chapters of this book, suggestions will be found for the adaptation and modification of equipment. These are intended to overcome some of the difficulties disabled people find in handling normal equipment. A simple modification to a fishing rod may make casting or control easier. Taping on a mark where the hand grips the paddle will enable a blind canoeist to gauge the angle of entry of the blade into the water. A back rest in the canoe may ease the sitting position of a person who has lost the use of his legs. The use of a sling can open up exciting possibilities for a one-armed water skier. There are other adaptations which have been successfully tried, but some have been rejected because they were too clumsy, or added to the danger. Although experiments continue, instructors are frequently surprised at the ingenuity of disabled people themselves in finding ways to handle ordinary equipment. It cannot be stressed too strongly that, as far as possible, it is best to use the normal equipment and to make modifications only when they are necessary. If this is done, clubs are often willing to loan equipment in the early stages to get things started. It is wise not to buy personal equipment until it has been thoroughly tested as suitable for the particular disability.

Equipment is expensive but sometimes costs can be reduced by making one's own. Adult education classes in boat and canoe building, and in fly-tying, are run in some areas. Visits to exhibitions can reveal the range of equipment available, and also show what some interested manufacturers have produced in the way of modifications for disabled people.

Further information on equipment may be obtained from the B.S.A.D. National Co-ordinator for Water Sports. He will also be pleased to advise on any particular problem which may be encountered (see Appendix 4, p.250).

23. Guidance for Course Organisers

COURSES FOR INSTRUCTORS

There is a great need for people who already take part in a water sport and are prepared to learn about the special techniques required to allow disabled people to enjoy it. In the first instance courses should concern themselves with those having physical or sensory handicaps. As experience is gained, however, and with the advice of people working professionally in this field, it is hoped that courses will be directed towards the mentally handicapped also.

The Water Sports Division should be contacted about course proposals, and offers the following advice and suggestions to those running 'conversion' courses.

ORGANISATION

The time of year

A weekend in the spring or summer, probably Friday evening to Sunday afternoon, has been found to be most suitable. Off-peak times in the winter months should be avoided.

Place

A centre or club should be chosen where the staff or members are keen to welcome disabled people. Access to and within the premises, to the water's edge and from the car park, should all be considered before a decision is made. The choice of activities will depend partly on the demand but also on the provision available. Some activities such as sailing, canoeing and angling can be held together, whereas rowing, water skiing and sub-aqua will require special facilities.

Recruitment

If possible there should be a co-ordinator for each activity who will not only be able to instruct, but will also visit the site in advance and try out equipment etc. Course members should preferably be qualified instructors in the sport who wish to learn about teaching disabled people. They may be recruited from clubs, B.S.A.D. regions, the Regional Councils for Sport and Recreation or their water recreation committees, governing-body coaching associations, etc. Personal contact is generally the most successful.

It is essential to have disabled people as practice pupils and with as wide a variety of disabilities as possible — e.g. in wheelchairs, ambulant, blind, etc. They should be confident in cold water and it may be necessary to give a swimming test beforehand. They should be sufficient in number for all the instructors to have experience of dealing with a variety of handicaps. B.S.A.D. branches, special schools, swimming clubs for the disabled, and P.H.A.B. clubs, as well as personal contact, will help to find them.

Planning

Planning for the course should start months in advance. The co-operation of the centre or club and local association should be sought to share the work. Arrangements will need to be made for accommodation and transport as well as for application forms and medical consent forms for the disabled pupils and for any disabled instructors. It is very helpful to have someone who knows the disabled pupils and their medical needs, possibly a physical education teacher or physiotherapist.

The question of insurance, both for the individuals and for the course venue, should be examined (see pp.211 – 212).

Facilities

Access should be checked very carefully, preferably by asking someone in a wheelchair to go over the building and the activity areas. The accommodation, toilet and washing facilities and the social amenities should be included. It may be necessary to decide on the number of wheelchairs that can be accommodated.

The fire precautions should be examined, and if necessary the advice of the Fire Officer sought.

Equipment

A decision will be required on the boats, canoes etc. to be used and the modifications, if any, which will be necessary. Different types of lifejackets and buoyancy aids should be available, as well as wet suits and plenty of warm clothing. Blankets should be on hand for people leaving the water.

Programme

The following sessions have been found useful and successful:

1. Introductory talk on the purpose of the course; the place of water sports for the disabled; attitude towards integration; the role of the governing bodies of sport and of the Water Sports Division of B.S.A.D.
2. Talk/demonstration on lifting and handling disabled people. This should be given by a therapist and be very basic, aimed at those who have no experience of wheeling chairs and lifting people.
3. Group theory session by co-ordinators before going on the water.
4. Talk on the medical aspects; the more common disabilities and their relevance to water sports. The special needs of the blind and/or the deaf may merit a separate talk.
5. Clothing and equipment with special problems of the disabled.
6. Practical sessions on the water. Plenty of time should be allowed for these.
7. Other topics for discussion will include:
   other water sports
   governing-body proficiency awards and help
   club structure
   the importance of swimming
   establishing contacts.
8. The final session should allow ample time for discussion, questions and exchange of information.

COURSES FOR DISABLED PEOPLE

With a body of trained instructors, the task of introducing disabled people to water activities can be undertaken with confidence in an organised way. It will be necessary to follow the same careful advice as given above in selecting the venue, checking facilities, equipment and insurance. Early planning in all its detail will again be essential, and the help of other associations and bodies should be sought.

The pupil/instructor ratio may well be higher than for able-bodied people, and extra helpers who should be briefed well in advance will be needed.

If planning is careful there should be few problems. A person who knows the course members can help to allay any natural anxiety and apprehension which the centre staff or club members may feel. A sense of humour can overcome many difficulties, and disabled people will generally know what they need and when.

The programme should be flexible enough to cater for the varying physical abilities and stamina of members. Films can be incorporated at short notice, visits arranged and lectures given. The task is perhaps to strike the right balance between the two extremes of needlessly denying participants activities which are within their capabilities, and of encouraging them to believe they can manage activities beyond them. Successful achievement in the face of worthwhile challenge should be the keynote.

FOLLOW-UP

This is one of the most important aspects of any course. It should be ensured that both potential instructors and disabled people know what opportunities exist to teach or practise their sport. Once the introduction is made, the effort should not be wasted through lack of knowledge or failure to continue encouragement.

24. If You Want to Help

ADVICE TO TEACHERS AND OTHERS

Educational policy now encourages the integration of the handicapped into ordinary schools, but their inclusion in outdoor pursuits does not always follow as a matter of course. Unfortunately some disabled youngsters have become conditioned to watching their able-bodied friends enjoying activities without thinking of taking part themselves. The suggestion that they should do so may come as a pleasant surprise. Naturally there should be a check first that it would not be medically unwise, and also that it will be possible to meet the safety requirements of the sport, particularly with respect to confidence in cold water.

There is no need to be a teacher to become involved in teaching disabled pupils to sail, row, canoe or water ski. Some of those who are most active and skilled in this sphere are not professional teachers at all, but enthusiasts who have found that their offers of expert help have been readily accepted, especially if they have shown a knack for getting on well with children.

Training sessions should proceed in the usual manner with provision for helping handicapped members of the group to overcome any mobility problems, such as getting in and out of small craft, or up and down steps. Integrated activities usually prove highly successful because each person assists the other and there is plenty of help available. Often the disciplined approach and co-operative attitude of disabled youngsters has proved a valuable asset during weekend and holiday courses. The reluctance to include them has proved ill-founded.

The introduction of water sports activities in special schools for children of mixed disabilities will depend largely on the enthusiasm and expertise of the school staff. Where this step has been taken the result has not only been the obvious enjoyment that the activity has provided, but also a growth in confidence and an increased sense of responsibility. Frequently, however, school staff are hesitant to embark on a project for which they lack the expert knowledge, and in the face of what appear to be insurmountable difficulties. It is here that external instructors can provide the necessary help and establish the link between the school and club or regional training facilities. They may assist the school staff in sports sessions or they may undertake to organise short introductory courses, followed by further sessions for the more enthusiastic pupils.

It has been found that while those with a mental handicap should attend sessions which are specially arranged for them, there is little point in dividing physically handicapped classes into sub-groups consisting of individuals with similar disabilities. It is better to have ambulant and non-ambulant pupils paired off. Among the most successful combinations have been the visually handicapped working with the physically disabled.

It may be difficult to find lifejackets, buoyancy aids and safety helmets to fit those whose bodies and limbs are not of standard proportions. In such cases adaptation may be necessary, but care must be taken to ensure that fastenings and fittings stay in the intended position, and that the equipment will function correctly. If leg irons or calipers must be worn they should be included in the total weight to be supported in the water by the buoyancy equipment. Caliper wearers should not be on the water by themselves because of the difficulty they may experience in extracting themselves from capsized canoes or dinghies.

Special care must be taken to ensure that pupils are not subject to exposure. Protective clothing of the right kind, as described elsewhere in this book (pp.204 and 246), will be particularly important, and there should be alertness for any signs of reduction in stamina or early indications of hypothermia.

As the pupils leave schools, and in courses for adult disabled groups, the aim should clearly be eventual integration into local club activities. 'Non-integrated' taster courses can familiarise the disabled person with the difficulties he is likely to encounter, and provide him with the opportunity to solve some of the most immediate problems in private. The task of the teacher or instructor will be to ease the transition by establishing links with clubs and by giving advice on follow-up. Further repeat courses will be arranged for the more severely handicapped who would find difficulty in joining a club, but it is hoped that the others will be able to enjoy their sport in the company of their able-bodied fellows.

25. Handling and Manoeuvring a Disabled Person

As a result of the development of water sports for the disabled, many able-bodied people are coming into contact with disabled people for the first time, and encountering unfamiliar situations. Lack of knowledge of how to give assistance may cause confusion, embarrassment, and injury to the helper or the 'helped', or to both of them.

Obviously, it is impossible to describe in a few pages how to cope with every disability in every situation. However, by remembering a few simple rules, most problems can be overcome.

Let us first consider what is meant by 'disabled'. Depending on their mobility problems, disabled people may be placed into four broad categories.

1. *Non-ambulant*

This group consists of those who spend most of their lives in wheel-chairs. However, some of them may be able to walk a few paces or stand for short periods of time.

2. *Ambulant disabled*

This group is made up of those who need the assistance of any walking aid or appliance to assist their mobility. These include sticks, crutches, frames, calipers and artificial limbs.

3. *Ambulant but requiring manual assistance*

Included in this group are those who can perhaps normally manage to walk alone, and to manoeuvre quite safely on normal firm surfaces, but with unknown factors involved in jetties, slipways, pontoons etc. may need the assistance of one or more people to manage with safety. A steadying hand may be all that is necessary.

4. *Blind and partially sighted*

Although this group have no physical mobility problems, they will naturally need considerable assistance in negotiating the unknown. Verbal explanations need to be extra clear, and physical assistance as guidance will be needed to help them to avoid hazards, especially in the early stages. It should be remembered that every disabled person is an individual and will have different requirements. Even those with similar disabilities may not need the same kind of help. It is always prudent to ask the disabled person directly how he can best be helped.

LIFTING THE DISABLED

In considering how to 'lift' someone a feat of great strength is not supposed. It is rather a planned pattern of movement in which the helper or helpers and the disabled can work as a team.

To be able to plan and carry out the pattern of movement to transfer a disabled person, for example, from a wheelchair to a boat, without harm to the disabled or the helpers, some understanding of basic anatomy and body mechanics will be helpful.

Basic anatomy

The spinal column of the body is made up of twenty-four bones called *vertebrae*. Between each vertebra is a disc which acts as a shock absorber. Each vertebra is supported by ligaments and muscles. This bony spinal

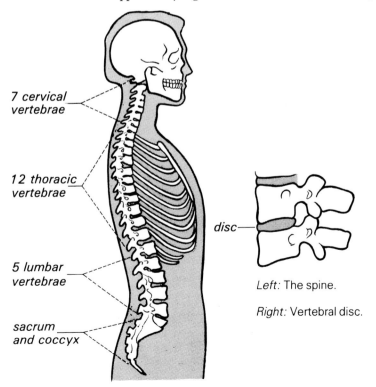

7 cervical vertebrae

12 thoracic vertebrae

5 lumbar vertebrae

sacrum and coccyx

disc—

Left: The spine.

Right: Vertebral disc.

column protects the vital spinal cord and allows the individual nerves to pass from the spinal cord to supply the arms and legs and other parts of the body. Keeping the trunk as straight as possible during any lifting action will minimise the strain on the spine. Damage to the ligaments, muscles and discs will lead to severe pain and discomfort.

Use the strongest muscles

The greater part of the work of lifting should be done by the legs, the muscles of which are very strong in comparison with those of the spine. In preparing for the lift the legs should be bent in a relaxed manner, thus lowering the body. This will bring the arms into the correct position for lifting. Balance will be retained and the top-heavy forward-leaning movement of the trunk avoided. This is a common fault in inexpert lifting. Correct posture will enable the legs and arms to be used without strain on the back. No more energy than necessary will be exerted.

Make sure that the effort is correctly directed

The helper's feet should be placed in the direction of movement, so that the helper and the 'helped' move as a combined unit. Handling the disabled must be:

1. safe
2. comfortable
3. adequate
4. appropriate
5. unobtrusive
6. not excessive

Safe

In establishing the safest method of handling, guidance must be sought from the disabled person. He will know his own abilities and limitations, and particularly at the beginning, his wishes must be closely followed. The helper must ask him how he prefers to be moved. An element of trust and security will be built up, and if time is taken at the beginning, anxiety may be avoided.

Comfortable

If either party is uncomfortable, the lift is in danger of becoming unsafe and awkward. If there is any doubt, the movement should be started again and the uncomfortable component changed, whether it be grip, stance or whatever.

Adequate and appropriate but not excessive

This again depends on what is required by the individual, and this is why it is so important to ask first. If the assistance is not adequate or is excessive, fear could develop, making future handling more difficult.

Unobtrusive

Disabled people wish to be considered as normal as possible, and it is therefore vitally important that any help be given as unobtrusively as possible. This avoids drawing attention to the individual, and consequent embarrassment. If any manoeuvre is causing problems to either party, one solution

Helping a young disabled person from a wheelchair. She sits well forward. The lifter stands close with straight back, front knee bent and wide stance. The hand grip is under one arm and round the shoulders.

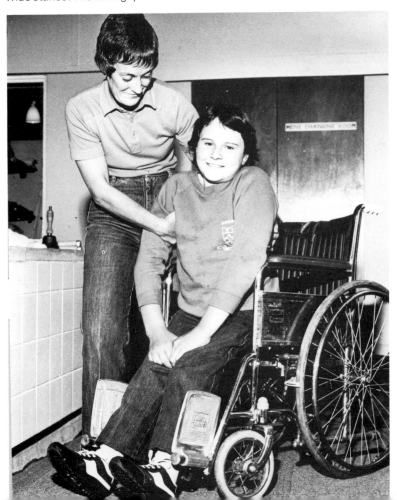

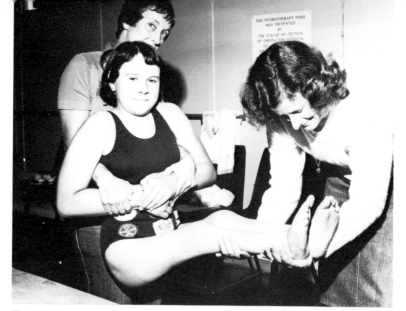

The lifter at rear has through arm grasp and stands very close. The second helper supports and lifts the legs.

is for the helper to mimic the disability and the situation. In this way a satisfactory solution may be found, and the disabled person and helper can decide on the preferred procedure. As in most situations, a sense of humour helps!

Being lowered into the water. The helper on the right stands close and has a comfortable grasp under the arms. She keeps the back straight, the legs doing all the work. The disabled child supports herself on the second helper's shoulders.

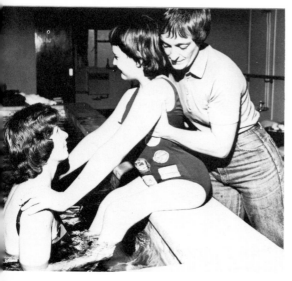

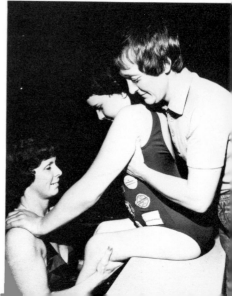

Basic points of lifting

When lifting or manoeuvring a disabled person, it is important to remember the following points:

1. Keep as close as possible to the disabled person during the movement. This will ensure that it is the legs and strong trunk muscles that are doing the work, and not the arms or weaker spinal joints and muscles that take the strain.
2. Get a good, firm comfortable grip.

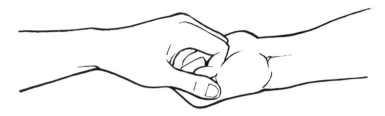

The finger grasp: a longer reach but the nails must be kept short.

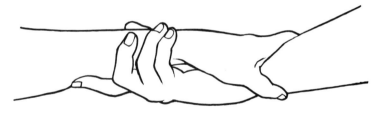

The double wrist grasp. A single grasp is used when the disabled person is too weak to grip.

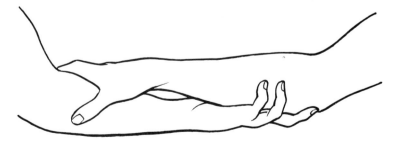

The double forearm grasp.

3.   The feet should be pointing in the direction of travel.
4.   A disabled person's limbs might involuntarily give way; it is therefore essential that they be properly supported during the lift.

When lifting, bend the knees and hips and keep the back straight. Place the feet either level and a little way apart, or with one foot in front of the other, whichever way is more comfortable. Points 1 – 4 should be remembered before carrying out the lifting. Obviously it is not possible to include comprehensive instructions for all situations. For those dealing with a variety of different disabled people the following publications are recommended: *Handling the Handicapped* (Chartered Society of Physiotherapy), and *Safer Lifting for Patient Care*, Margaret Hollis (Blackwell Scientific Publications).

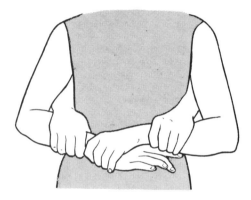

The through arm grasp. The disabled person grips one wrist with the other hand.

Points to guard against

A disabled person who is paralysed, or has loss of sensation or circulatory problems, is very prone to bruising, pressure abrasions, chafing and other skin damage, as he cannot feel pain in the affected parts. It is therefore necessary to provide extra protection to the vulnerable parts of the trunk, buttocks and legs.

There is also a greater chance than usual of the onset of hypothermia, as heat loss may go undetected. Again, adequate protective clothing is necessary.

However it is very important to guard against the impression of over-protecting the disabled person. If he requires help he will ask for it. It is also important to remember that if he has paralysed or damaged lower limbs, he

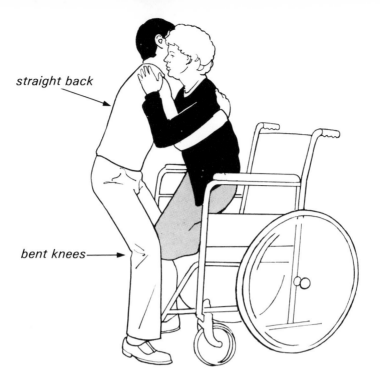

straight back

bent knees

Good position for one helper to lift a disabled person from a wheelchair.

Good position for two helpers to lift a disabled person from a wheelchair.

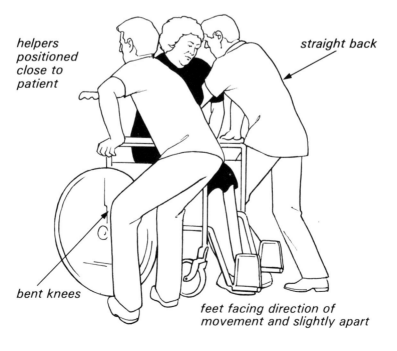

helpers positioned close to patient

straight back

bent knees

feet facing direction of movement and slightly apart

will usually have compensated by developing exceedingly strong upper limbs, which will enable him to carry out many activities using his arms only.

As long as these precautions are adhered to, water sports can be extremely enjoyable both for the instructor and the disabled person. However, when in doubt remember the golden rule: 'Ask the disabled person first.'

26. Hopes for the Future

The first edition of this handbook appeared in 1977, and it is now encouraging to look back and note the considerable progress which has since been made. The examples described of enjoyment of water sports by disabled people are only a small number among those known. It is heartening to think that there are many more, and that participation is increasing. More clubs and centres have opened their doors, while local authorities have become more acutely aware of their responsibilities.

However, there still remains a great deal to be done, and there is a need to work towards a situation in which disabled people will be able to use recreational facilities with the same ease and lack of restraint as the able-bodied.

Access

This is still a long way off, and the elimination of access problems must be the first priority. There are regrettably many public places from which disabled people are effectively barred because design has not taken account of their needs. Plenty of information is now available. New facilities must be planned with disabled access in mind, and existing centres must be converted to fulfil this requirement. Private clubs also need to look at their facilities and decide what their policy should be towards providing for disabled users. Perhaps it is a sign of things to come that in marina car parks it is now possible to find special places reserved for disabled drivers.

Techniques

Perhaps the greatest advances have been made in technical expertise. As the various sections of this handbook illustrate, there is now a wealth of material and simple modifications of equipment which instructors have devised to aid them in teaching the disabled. The Water Sports Division has collated this over the past few years and is very ready to supply information and to give advice. It is always glad to hear of new methods or techniques which have been evolved.

Training

There is a need for training at all levels, from the novice's first experience to the special teaching skills required by the instructors who take courses for the disabled. Only through well-organised and appropriate training will the safety and enjoyment of disabled water sports enthusiasts be ensured. Recognised proficiency awards in the various sports will provide an incentive for disabled and able-bodied alike. A time should come, however, when governing bodies will include, as a matter of course, a 'techniques for use with disabled people' option in their training syllabuses for instructors. The changes in attitude which have become apparent are to be welcomed, and this should be a continuing process.

Integration

Where progress has been greatest, however, it has often been because disabled enthusiasts have taken the initiative. Meeting their able-bodied counterparts more than half way, they have been able to convince them that the difficulties of integration can be overcome, and that advantages can accrue to both sides. Full integration of the disabled into society should be the eventual aim. Undoubtedly the best ambassadors are disabled people themselves. Perhaps the time is ripe for the governing bodies to consider whether they should now be appointing qualified and competent disabled representatives to undertake liaison with parents, schools and all who are concerned with outdoor education.

THE WATER SPORTS DIVISION

As for the Water Sports Division itself, its members have welcomed their incorporation into the wider structure of the British Sports Association for the Disabled which will lead to a new phase of development. The work within the committee has always been lively. The shared experience and closer liaison between the various water sports and the other bodies represented, which it has made possible, have been a continual stimulus.

International co-operation

Co-operation with similar groups and individuals working with disabled people in other countries has been a particularly rewarding experience. The International Seminar on Water Sports for Disabled People, organised in conjunction with the Sports Council as part of the I.Y.D.P. campaign in September 1981 (see Appendix 1), brought together much information and expertise from a number of countries. It fostered happy relationships which have since led to fruitful exchanges of visits and ideas.

There is obviously much to be gained from international pooling of experience of this kind. Varying lines of development have sometimes been followed in different countries. In Britain the emphasis has been on making existing and new facilities available for disabled and able-bodied alike, and on the integration of the disabled into normal clubs. Elsewhere centres have been established where the emphasis has been on catering for the disabled, and staff with a medical or therapeutic background have been appointed. Both approaches have much to offer and to learn from each other and are not necessarily mutually exclusive.

The recommendations made during the final session of the Seminar represent an ambitious programme, but the Water Sports Division will work towards their full implementation.

The welcome which the first handbook received, both in Britain and internationally, made it very evident that it had filled a need for guidance in an area where there were many who were eager to participate, but lacked the knowledge, and often the confidence to do so. This revised and much enlarged handbook is the fruit of further years of experience in which much has been learned. If it gives some idea of what can be achieved where the will exists, and makes it possible for others to share these exciting and rewarding recreational pursuits, it will have achieved its purpose.

Appendix 1. International Seminar on Water Sports for Disabled People, Nottingham, 1981

This seminar was one of the major events of the campaign of the Sports Councils of the United Kingdom 'Sport for All — Disabled People' in the International Year for the Disabled. It was organised in conjunction with the Water Sports Division of the British Sports Association for the Disabled.

The purpose of the seminar was to provide opportunities for more disabled people to take part in the water sports of their choice by exchanging and sharing information, expertise and ideas and considering ways and means for future co-operation and development.

Fifty-two delegates from nine countries (England, Wales, Scotland, U.S.A., France, Australia, Belgium, Northern Ireland, Norway) attended. Many of these were coaches and instructors. More than a dozen were themselves disabled water sports enthusiasts.

PROGRAMME

The programme covered the six main water sports of sailing, canoeing, angling, water skiing, sub-aqua and rowing.

Papers were given on the following topics:

- Medical Considerations
- Water Sports and People with Mental Handicap
- Developments Around the World
    Accounts were given of progress in individual sports by
    representatives of the various countries.
- Teaching methods and the Role of Teachers
- The Role of the Therapist
- Facilities and Organisations
- Survival, Scientific aspects and clothing design.

Some time was also devoted to practical demonstrations in which new equipment, craft, and adaptations were used, and there was also an opportunity for participation by delegates.

RECOMMENDATIONS

The following recommendations were agreed and forwarded to the Council of Europe Committee for the Development of Sport, which supported the seminar. It is hoped that action on them will be taken within the individual countries represented.

1. Each country should establish a focal point for collecting, holding and disseminating information relating to bibliography, courses, seminars and equipment.
2. The national governing bodies of water sports should ultimately assume responsibility for disabled people within their sports. This would involve the training of coaches, instructors and officials and, through member clubs, the integration of disabled people into the sport wherever appropriate.
3. International sports federations should similarly assume responsibility at international level.
4. Disabled sports organisations, in close liaison with governing bodies, should, as part of their co-ordinating role, encourage people with disabilities to participate in water sports.
5. Each country should ensure that every opportunity is provided to encourage those people with disabilities who so wish to take part in the water sport(s) of their choice. This would include the involvement of statutory, professional and voluntary organisations concerned with education, sport, welfare, youth, disability and rehabilitation. Particular stress should be placed on persuading the medical profession of the value of water sports to disabled people.
6. Specific attention should be given to the relatively new development of water sports with mentally handicapped people. Their problems are different from those of the physically and sensorily handicapped and may require different solutions.
7. While the emphasis should remain on the broad development of water sports as recreation, the place of competition, wherever appropriate, should be considered.
8. Another international seminar should be held within two years.
9. In the mean time, there should be regular exchanges of information between countries, and encouragement should be given to other countries to develop water sports with disabled people.

Appendix 2. Making Clothing Yourself

MAKING AN ANORAK

A pattern for making an anorak is given below. Cut a full-size pattern using newspaper or other big sheets of paper. The anorak needs to be roomy to help ventilation and to allow extra woollens to be worn underneath. The sizes given are without seam allowance, so a good inch extra needs to be added where shown. The pattern always looks too big!

Cutting out

Anyone who has only a little experience of sewing should make a trial garment using an old sheet or other old material. Remember to check that the pattern is lying on the correct side of your fabric.

Sewing

Use a big stitch with as little tension as possible. As the only difficult part is the hood, it is suggested this be done first. With right sides together sew from P to K, so that when turned inside out the hood shape is made.

A pattern for making an anorak.

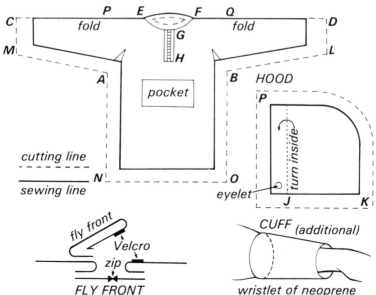

On the main anorak piece cut the neck hole as shown and slit G – H for the zip. Turn this piece inside out.

Pin the hood in the neck hole starting at centre back so that J ends half an inch in from the slit (G – H) for the zip. This gives half an inch turn-in for the zip hem, and the hood turns inside to form the tunnel for the draw-cord. This tunnel will be sewn after the zip has been put in.

Put an eyelet each side for the draw cord exits. Turn back the half-inch side of slit G – H and put in the zip.

If a pocket is wanted it should be sewn in now. Make a model of the pocket in paper first.

Sew a flap above the pocket. Add 'velcro' tape to keep the flap shut.

Sew L – B – O and M – A – N.

Now hem the sleeves and the bottom edge of the anorak to the required length.

The garment is now complete.

If the anorak looks 'wingy' under the arm, a dart back and front, as shown in the diagram, will cure this tendency. Sew the darts before sewing the side seams.

Seams

Any seam is better than a simple seam (e.g. french seam). To proof the seam put on Bostik No. 1 or Bostik 3206 which is used in making up diving wet suits.

Zipped jacket

If a zipped jacket is preferred, the slit G – H can be extended to the bottom of the garment and an open-ended zip put in. A full length 'fly' is then necessary.

High trousers

If a fly is not included, trousers are very easy to make. The pattern is simply two halves with crutch and side seams only (Diagram p.248). The trousers are high-waisted, coming to roughly below the armpits. They can be cut out like normal trousers and the high waist added later, if this is easier.

Two pieces of similar shape should be cut. The seam A – B – C will be the centre front and E – D – C will be the centre back. These seams need to be very strong, preferably taped for strength and waterproofing. Join sides J – K – L to G – H – I.

If there are dressing problems, a lightweight open-ended zip could be put down these seams (i.e. down each outside leg).

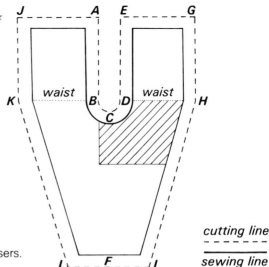

A guide to making high trousers.
C – F inside leg
B – C – D waist front, under crutch to waist back
L – I size round trouser bottom (leg)
A – B, D – E waist to armpit

A strip of fabric, or loops sewn on at the waist, are suitable for a draw cord. A large hem around the top of the trousers provides a tunnel for a draw cord under the arms.

Two pieces of the same shape as the shaded area can be cut out and put in to provide a double seat.

The best pattern is an old pair of trousers that fit comfortably, opened into two pieces as shown. It should be remembered that waterproof trousers need to be on the large side as they will be worn over other trousers.

MATERIALS

Clothing worn by those taking part in water sports needs to be windproof and waterproof. All modern waterproof fabrics will also be windproof, but they tend to suffer from condensation. A fabric which is too thin should not be used as the proofing may soon wear away.

A 4oz/sq.yd fabric is advised for wear and strength. This will normally have a layer of polyurethane (P.U.) on the inside to provide the waterproofing. A silicone spray applied on the outside will make the water run off more easily. If thinner fabrics only are available, two layers should be used, particularly over the shoulders and back.

Where a group of people intend making a number of garments it might be much cheaper to purchase a roll of fabric directly from the manufacturers.

Appendix 3. Medical Form

This form should be filled in and signed by a doctor, or completed by a therapist who knows the applicant and signed by a doctor.

THE COURSE AND THE CENTRE

Give information, for guidance of the person filling in the form, on type of building, availability of medical support, activities to be undertaken, proposed daily programme, staffing available, what is required of students etc:

_____

_____

_____

_____

_____

1. Name

_____

2. Address

_____

_____

_____Age_____

3. Swimming ability

_____

4. Diagnosis

_____

_____

5. Any additional handicap(s)

_____

_____

_____

6. Drugs in use

_____

_____

_____

7. Allergies

_____

_____

8. Does the applicant suffer from:
(a) Epilepsy? If so, please give details of severity and control

_____

_____

(b) Diabetes?

_____

_____

9. Please indicate applicant's degree of mobility

☐ Ambulant (please state roughly over what distance on footpaths):

☐ Ambulant over short distances and uses wheelchair

☐ Mobile only in wheelchair

10. Those filling in this form are asked to use their discretion in mentioning such topics as age, temperament, eyesight, hearing, speech impairment, incontinence, appliances worn, ability to use stairs, which may have special relevance to centre staff:

_____

_____

_____

This applicant is, in my opinion, fit to attend the course described above

Doctor's signature

_____

Address

_____

Appendix 4. Addresses, Bibliography and Films

ADDRESSES

The Sports Council, 16 Upper Woburn Place, London WC1H 0QP

Amateur Swimming Association, Harold Fern House, Derby Square, Loughborough, Leics. LE11 0AL, Tel: 0509 30431

Amateur Rowing Association, 6 Lower Mall, London W6 9DJ, Tel: 01-748 3632

British Canoe Union, Flexel House, 45-47 High Street, Addlestone, Weybridge, Surrey KT15 1JV, Tel: Weybridge 41341

British Sub-Aqua Club, 16 Upper Woburn Place, London WC1H 0QW, Tel: 01-387 9302

British Water Ski Federation, 16 Upper Woburn Place, London WC1H 0QL, Tel: 01-387 9371

National Anglers' Council, 11 Cowgate, Peterborough, Cambs. PE1 1LZ, Tel: 0735 54084

Royal Yachting Association, Victoria Way, Woking, Surrey GU21 1EQ, Tel: 04862 5022

Model Yachting Association, 6 Rowner Close, Rowner, Gosport, Hants.

Model Power Boat Association, 36 Broadmeads, Ware, Herts.

Organisations for the Disabled

British Sports Association for the Disabled, Ludwig Guttmann Sports Centre — Stoke Mandeville, Harvey Road, Aylesbury, Bucks. HP21 8PP, Tel: 0296 27889

B.S.A.D. Water Sports Division, National Co-ordinator, Mr L. D. Warren, 29 Ironlatch Avenue, St Leonard's-on-Sea, East Sussex TN39 9JE, Tel: 0424 427931

Scottish Sports Association for the Disabled, c/o Scottish Sports Council, 1 St Colme Street, Edinburgh EH3 6AA, Tel: 031-225 8411

Welsh Sports Association for the Disabled, Mrs E. Roberts, Crosswinds, 14 Cae Gam, Heol-y-Cyw, Bridgend, Mid-Glamorgan, Tel: 0656 860854

Sports Council for Northern Ireland, 2A Upper Malone Road, Belfast BT9 5LA, Tel: 0232 663154

British Disabled Water Ski Association, Warren Wood, The Warren, Ashtead, Surrey KT21 2SN

The Bluebird Deaf Water Ski Club, Sec. Mr A. M. Thomas, 63 Runton Road, Cromer, Norfolk.

Association of Swimming Therapy, Treetops, Malpas Road, Tilston Malpas, Cheshire SY14 7HL

National Association of Swimming Clubs for the Handicapped, 63, Dunvegan Road, Eltham, London SE9

R.Y.A. Seamanship Foundation, Victoria Way, Woking, Surrey GU21 1EQ

Disabled Living Foundation, 346 Kensington High Street, London W14 8NS

Royal Association for Disability and Rehabilitation (R.A.D.A.R.), 25, Mortimer Street, London W1N 8AB. (Apply to the Holiday Officer for *Sparkle* bookings.)

Rocky Mountain Spinal Injury Center Inc., Craig Hospital, 3425 South Clarkson, Englewood, Colorado, U.S.A.

National Association of Underwater Instructors (N.A.U.I.) (Canada), Box 510, Etobicoke, Ontario, Canada M9C 4V5

Handicapped Scuba Association, 1104 El Prado, San Clemente, CA 92672, U.S.A.

Vinland National Center, 3675 Ihduhapi Road, Loretto, Minnesota 55357 U.S.A.

Committee for Handicap Sailing, Baerum Seilforening, Strandalleen 8, 1320 Stabekk, Norway

Navisport, 3 avenue Guy de Larigaudie, B.P. 504, 44026 NANTES, Cedex, France

Other organisations

Countryside Commission, John Dower House, Crescent Place, Cheltenham, Glos. GL50 3RA

Water Space Amenity Commission, 1 Queen Anne's Gate, London SW1H 9BT, Tel: 01-222 8111

British Waterways Board, Melbury House, Melbury Terrace, London NW1 6JX, Tel: 01-262 6711

Inland Waterways Association, 114 Regents Park Road, London NW1 8UQ, Tel: 01-586 2556

Marine Division of the Department of Trade, Sunley House, 90-93 High Holborn, London WC1V 6LP, Tel: 01-405 6911

National Yacht Harbour Association, Harleyford, Marlow, Bucks., Tel: 06284 71361

Ship and Boat Builders National Federation, Boating Industry House,
Vale Road, Oatlands Village, Weybridge, Surrey, Tel: Weybridge 54511
Yacht Charter Association, 33 Highfield Road, Lymington, Hants.
Royal National Lifeboat Institution, West Quay Road, Poole,
Dorset BH15 1HZ
British Standards Institution, 101 Pentonville Road, London N1 9ND
Jubilee Sailing Trust, Tavistock House North, Tavistock Square,
London WC1H 9HX
Peter Le Marchant Trust, Colston Bassett, Nottingham NG12 3FE
Heulwen-Sunshine, Mrs C. Millington, Green Acre, Salop Road, Welshpool,
Powys
Willow Wren Hire Cruises, Rugby Wharf, off Consul Road, Leicester Road,
Rugby
Seagull Trust, 1 Dirleton Road, North Berwick EH39 5BY
Midland Luxury Cruises Ltd, 19 Common Road, Evesham, Worcestershire
Blakes Broads Tours Ltd, Station Road, Wroxham, Norwich, Norfolk
The Calvert Trust, Adventure Centre for the Disabled, Little Crosthwaite,
Underskiddaw, Keswick, Cumbria

Suppliers

Raymond Sims Limited, 34 Hampton Road, West Bridgford, Nottingham
(The Playboat)
Buccleuch Engineering Ltd, Queen Ann Drive, Newbridge Industrial Estate,
Midlothian
Valley Canoe Products, Nottingham (The Caranoe)
P & H Fibreglass Productions, Derby (individual canoe modifications)

BIBLIOGRAPHY

General

Informal Countryside Recreation for Disabled People (Countryside
Commission)
Outdoor Pursuits for Disabled People Croucher (Woodhead Faulkner
Limited)
Physical Education for Special Needs Groves (Cambridge University Press)
Physical Education and the Handicapped Child Price
*Give us the Chance. Sport and physical recreation with mentally
handicapped people* (Disabled Living Foundation)

Water Sports and Epilepsy (Disability Studies Unit, Wildhanger, Amberley, Arundel, W. Sussex)

Safety in Outdoor Pursuits Department of Education and Science (HMSO, London)

Extension Activities Handbook (The Scout Association)

Holidays for the Handicapped (Royal Association for Disability and Rehabilitation)

Textbook of Sports for the Disabled Guttman (H M and M)

How to Contact Disabled People (Disabled Living Foundation)

Access and facilities

Designing for the Disabled Goldsmith (RIBA Publications)

Sports Facilities for Disabled People (Disabled Living Foundation)

Access for disabled people to buildings (British Standards Institution)

Water Safety

The following three titles are available from ROSPA, Cannon House, The Priory, Queensway, Birmingham B4 6BS:

On the Water, In the Water

Lifejackets and personal buoyancy aids

Cold Water can Kill

Drownproofing Bettsworth (Heinemann Educational Books, London)

INDIVIDUAL SPORTS

Angling

Guide to Fishing Facilities for the Disabled (National Anglers' Council)

Facilities for Disabled Anglers in Scotland (Scottish Sports Association for the Disabled)

Canoeing

Available from the British Canoe Union:

1   *Choosing a canoe and its equipment*
2   *Canoe handling and management*
7a *Canoe building — soft skin moulded veneer*
7b *Canoe building — glass fibre*
10 *Canoeing for the Disabled*

Sailing

Produced by the Royal Yachting Association:

Insurance in Yachting (910/75)

Flags and Signals (C4/76)
Weather Forecasts, Stations, Times etc. (95/75)
Addresses of National Authorities — R.Y.A.
 affiliated clubs and classes (913/76)
 Other sailing books listed in R.Y.A. catalogue:
The Sailing Manual Bob Bond
Learn to Sail
Going Afloat
Know the Game — Sailing (EP Publishing Ltd)
They Said We Couldn't Do It ed. Chartres (R.Y.A. Seamanship Foundation)
Boating for the Handicapped Hedley (Human Resources Center, Albertson, NY 11507 U.S.A.)
Open Boating: Water Safety and Boating for the Disabled Goldberg and Webel (City of Oakland, U.S.A.)

Water Skiing

Know the Game — Water Skiing (EP Publishing Ltd)
Water Skiing Athans and Ward (Collier Macmillan)
Additional Code of Practice for Disabled Water Skiers (British Disabled Water Ski Association)

Lifting and Handling

Handling the Handicapped Chartered Society of Physiotherapy (Woodhead Faulkner)
Safer Lifting for Patient Care Hollis (Blackwell)
Lifting and Handling National Co-ordinating Committee on Swimming for the Disabled (The Sports Council)

Swimming

Guidelines on Teaching Disabled People to Swim Trussell (Swimming Teachers Association)
The Teaching of Swimming (Amateur Swimming Association)
Swimming for the Disabled Association of Swimming Therapy (EP Publishing Ltd)

FILMS

Not Just a Spectator (Town and Country Productions, Cheyne Row, Chelsea, London)

Water Free (swimming) (Town and Country)

It's Ability that Counts (B.S.A.D.)

Riding towards Freedom Riding for the Disabled Association (Town and Country)

Able to Fish (series) (Town and Country)

    1. *Coarse Angling*

    2. *Game Fishing*

    3. *Sea Angling*

Breaking down the Barriers (Queensland, Australia) (Town and Country)

Give us the Chance. Activities for Mentally Handicapped People (Town and Country)

Free Dive Horus Productions (Available in the U.K. through the British Sub-Aqua Club)